Medical Statistics

Fiona Collen
Southampton
April 1993

Medical Statistics

A Commonsense Approach

MICHAEL J. CAMPBELL

Medical Statistics and Computing
University of Southampton

and

DAVID MACHIN

Medical Research Council Cancer Trials Office
Cambridge

JOHN WILEY & SONS
Chichester · New York · Brisbane · Toronto · Singapore

Distributed in the United States of America, Canada and Japan by Alan R. Liss Inc.,
41 East 11th Street, New York, NY 10003, USA.

Other Wiley Editorial Offices

John Wiley & Sons, Inc., 605 Third Avenue,
New York, NY 10158-0012, USA

Jacaranda Wiley Ltd, G.P.O. Box 859, Brisbane,
Queensland 4001, Australia

John Wiley & Sons (Canada) Ltd, 22 Worcester Road,
Rexdale, Ontario M9W 1L1, Canada

John Wiley & Sons (SEA) Pte Ltd, 37 Jalan Pemimpin 05-04,
Block B, Union Industrial Building, Singapore 2057

Library of Congress Cataloging-in-Publication Data:

Campbell, Michael J.
    Medical statistics : a commonsense approach / by Michael J.
Campbell and David Machin.
        p.   cm.
    Includes bibliographical references.
    ISBN 0 471 91881 4
    1. Medical statistics.   I. Machin, David.   II. Title.
    [DNLM: 1. Biometry—methods.   2. Research Design.   3. Statistics.
WA 950 C189m]
R853.S7C36   1989
610′.72—dc20
DNLM/DLC
for Library of Congress   89-22419
                                                                    CIP

British Library Cataloguing in Publication Data:

Campbell, Michael J. (Michael Joseph, *1950–*)
    Medical statistics : a common sense approach.
    1. Medicine. Statistical methods
    I. Title   II. Machin, David
    610′.28

    ISBN 0 471 91881 4

Printed in Great Britain by Courier International Ltd., Tiptree, Colchester.

To Jacinta and Chris

List of contents

Preface

It is widely acknowledged that the use of statistical thinking as expressed by what appears in the medical literature is generally poor. This is despite the fact that there are a large number of excellent statistical textbooks on the market at present. The trouble, as we see it, is that medical students, nurses and doctors are far too busy to wade their way through a large technical handbook to learn what is essentially quite a difficult subject. Luckily, personal computers and statistical software are now widely available, and so the technical details of how to actually do a statistical test are now less important than they were. However, software manuals are not statistical textbooks, and the ease with which much analysis can be done means that there is a great danger of techniques being wrongly applied. As a consequence we felt there was a need for a book which not only tells one which statistics to use to summarise data and the assumptions underlying certain statistical methods, but also, and perhaps more importantly, discusses what restrictions there are to using the methods and when not to use them.

A good analysis must be preceded by a good design. The design of studies is often not given sufficient emphasis in books on statistics, but as practising medical statisticians, we spend much more of our time giving advice on the design of studies than we do on the actual analysis. The chapters in this book follow approximately the order of the phases of a study. Thus the chapters on design precede the chapters on analysis.

Many clinicians are not actually producers of studies involving statistics, but almost all will be consumers. They must read the medical literature to keep up to date and there they will find many papers contain a good deal of statistical analysis. Thus each chapter in the book contains a section on 'Points when reading the literature'.

We hope that this book will prove useful to medical students and student nurses by providing a concise explanation of the underlying principles in medical statistics, while keeping techniques in the background. They should be able to differentiate between good and poor uses of statistics. We also hope that clinicians embarking on research might be guided to draw correct inferences from their studies by using efficient designs and valid statistics. All the examples in the book are drawn from the current medical literature, or are based on our own research.

We have included material not usually found in a medical statistics textbook, such as the interpretation of diagnostic tests, relative operating characteristic (ROC) curves, survival analysis, case-control and cohort studies. These areas are often referred to in the medical literature and so we felt merited inclusion. For example, clinicians often have to read descriptions of epidemiological studies and ask themselves whether the findings are applicable to their particular patients, and we hope that this book will help them in this.

Finally, we recognise that some people may not have access to statistical software, and so we provide an Appendix with the computational details of commonly used procedures which could be carried out on a calculator. We have included some useful, but perhaps slightly more advanced techniques in the Appendix, such as Normal probability plots, the log-rank test and sample size calculations.

We thank many people for comments on previous versions of this book, in particular Drs Wim Gorissen, Geoffrey Berry and David Coggon. We thank Lesley Brewster for drawing some of the figures, John Williams for computational help and Lindsey Izzard and Tina Perry for word-processing.

Chapter 1

Uses and abuses of medical statistics

Summary

Statistical analysis features in the majority of papers published in medical journals. Most medical practitioners will need a basic understanding of statistical principles, but not necessarily statistical techniques. Medical statistics can contribute to good research by improving the design of studies as well as suggesting the optimum analysis of the results. Medical statisticians should be consulted early in the planning of a study. They can contribute in a variety of ways at all stages and not just at the final analysis of the data once they have been collected.

1.1 INTRODUCTION

Most medical practitioners do not carry out medical research. However, if they pride themselves on being up to date then they will definitely be *consumers* of medical research. It is incumbent on them to be able to discern good studies from bad; to be able to verify whether the conclusions of a study are valid and to understand the limitations of such studies.

A particular example might be a paper describing the results of a clinical trial of a new drug. A physician might read this report to try to decide whether to use the drug on his or her own patients. Since physicians are responsible for the care of their patients, it is their own responsibility to ensure the validity of the report, and its possible generalisation to particular patients. Usually, in the reputable medical press, the reader is to some extent protected from grossly misleading papers by both specialist and statistical referees. However, often there is no such protection in the general press or in much of the promotional literature sponsored by self-interested parties. However, even in the medical literature, misleading results can get through the refereeing net and no journal offers a guarantee as to the validity of its papers.

The use of statistical methods pervades the medical literature. In a survey of original articles published in the *New England Journal of Medicine*, Emerson and Colditz (1983) found that 70% used some form of statistical analysis, and we have discovered similar proportions in the *British Medical Journal* and the *Lancet*. It appears, therefore, that the majority of papers published in these medical journals require some statistical knowledge for a complete understanding.

Statistics is not only a discipline in its own right but it is also a fundamental tool for investigation in all biological and medical science. As such, any serious investigator in these fields must have a grasp of the basic principles. With modern computer facilities there is little need for familiarity with the technical details of statistical calculations. However, a physician should understand when such calculations are valid, when they are not and how they should be interpreted.

1.2 WHY USE STATISTICS?

To students schooled in the 'hard' sciences of physics and chemistry it is difficult to appreciate the variability of biological data. If one repeatedly puts blue litmus paper into acid solutions it turns red 100% of the time, not most (say 95%) of the time.

Penicillin was perhaps one of the few 'miracle' cures where the results were so dramatic that little evaluation was required.

However, if one gives aspirin to a group of people with headaches, not all of them will experience relief.

Measurements on human subjects rarely give exactly the same results from one occasion to the next. For example, if one measures the blood pressure of an individual on one particular day to within 1 mmHg, the chances that a measurement made under identical conditions the next day is within 5 mmHg of the original value has been calculated as less than 50% (Armitage *et al.*, 1966).

This variability is also inherent in responses to biological hazards. Most people now accept that cigarette smoking causes lung cancer and heart disease, and yet nearly everyone can point to an apparently healthy 80-year-old who has smoked for sixty years without apparent ill effect.

Although up to 20% of deaths in Britain are attributable to smoking according to the Royal College of Physicians (1983), it is usually forgotten that until the 1950s, the cause of the rise in lung cancer deaths was a mystery and commonly associated with diesel fumes. It was not until the carefully designed and statistically analysed case-control and cohort studies of Doll and Hill (1964) and others, that smoking was identified as the true cause.

With such variability, it follows that in any comparison made in a medical context, differences are almost bound to occur. These differences may be due to real effects, random variation or both. It is the job of the analyst to decide how much variation should be ascribed to chance, so that any remaining variation can be assumed to be due to a real effect. This is the art of statistics.

1.3 STATISTICS IS ABOUT COMMON SENSE AND GOOD DESIGN

A well designed study, poorly analysed, can be rescued by a reanalysis but a poorly designed study is beyond the redemption of even sophisticated statistics. Many experimenters only consult the medical statistician at the end of the study when the data have been collected. They believe that the job of the statistician is simply to analyse the data, and with powerful computers available, even complex studies with many variables can be easily processed. However, analysis is only part of a statistician's job, and calculation of the final 'p-value' a minor one at that!

A far more important task for the medical statistician is to ensure that results are comparable and generalisable. As an example, consider a study conducted by Burke and Yiamouyannis (1975) on the relation between cancer mortality and fluoridation of water supplies. Here fluoride in the drinking water is termed the *exposure* variable and cancer mortality the *outcome* variable. They considered 10 fluoridated and 10 non-fluoridated towns in the USA.

In the fluoridated towns, the cancer mortality rate had increased by 20% between 1950 and 1970, whereas in the non-fluoridated towns the increase was only 10%. From this they concluded that fluoridisation caused cancer. However, Oldham and Newell (1977), in a careful analysis of the age–sex–race structure of the 20 cities in 1950 and 1970, showed that in fact the excess cancer rate in the fluoridated cities increased by 1% over the 20 years, and in the non-fluoridated cities the increase was 4%. They concluded from this that there was no evidence that fluoridisation caused cancer. No statistical significance testing was deemed necessary by these authors, both medical statisticians, even though the paper appeared in a statistical journal!

In this example age, sex and race are examples of *confounding* variables. Any observational study that compares populations distinguished by a particular variable (such as a comparison of smokers and non-smokers) and ascribes the differences found in other variables (such as lung cancer rates) to that particular one is open to the charge that the observed differences are in fact due to some other, confounding, variables. Thus, the difference in lung cancer rates between smokers and non-smokers has been ascribed to genetic factors; that is, some factor that makes people want to smoke also makes them more susceptible to lung cancer. The difficulty with observational studies is that there is an infinite source of potential confounding variables. An investigator can measure all the variables that seem reasonable to him but a critic can always think of another, unmeasured, variable that just might explain the result. It is only in *randomised* studies that this logical difficulty is avoided. In randomised studies, where exposure variables (such as alternative treatments) are assigned purely by a chance mechanism, it can be assumed that unmeasured confounding variables are comparable, on average, in the two groups. Unfortunately, in many circumstances it is not possible to randomise the exposure variable, as in the case of smoking and lung cancer, and so alternative interpretations are always possible.

1.4 HOW A STATISTICIAN CAN HELP

Statistical ideas relevant to good design and analysis are difficult and we would always advise an investigator to seek the advice of a statistician at an early stage of an investigation. Here are some ways the medical statistician might help.

(a) Sample size and power considerations

One of the commonest questions asked of a consulting statistician is: How large should my study be? If the investigator has a reasonable amount of knowledge as to the likely outcome of a study, and potentially large resources of finance and time, then the statistician has mathematical tools available to enable a scientific answer to be made to the question. However, the usual scenario is that the investigator has either a grant of a limited size, or limited time, or a limited pool of patients. Nevertheless, given certain assumptions the medical statistician is still able to help. For a given number of patients the probability of obtaining effects of a certain size can be calculated. If the outcome variable is simply success or failure, the statistician will need to know the expected percentage of successes in each group. If the outcome variable is a quantitative measurement, it will be necessary to know the expected size of the difference between the two groups, and the variability of the measurement. For example, in a survey to see if patients with diabetes have raised blood pressure the medical statistician might say, 'with 100 diabetics and 100 healthy subjects in this survey and a possible difference in blood pressure of 5 mmHg, with standard deviation 10 mmHg, you have a 20% chance of obtaining a statistically significant result at the 5% level'. This means that one would anticipate that in only 1 trial in 5 of the proposed size would a statistically significant result be obtained. The investigator would then have to decide whether it was sensible or ethical to conduct a trial with such a small probability of success. One option would be to increase the size of the survey until success (defined as a statistically significant result when a difference of 5 mmHg does exist) becomes more probable.

(b) Questionnaires

Medical statisticians often have much experience in designing questionnaires, particularly so that they can be easily coded for computer analysis. Computers deal more efficiently with answers to questions that are in 'closed' form, that is where there is a limited number of replies allowed, but it is clearly important that the range of replies allowed covers the responses adequately.

It can be a very time-consuming task 'coding' a questionnaire, that is translating replies into numerical codes. Some questionnaires can be 'self-coded' in that the answer codes are printed with the question and then they can be entered directly into the computer. Other simple advice would include that, for example, it is usually better to have a separate code for 'missing', rather than leave the space blank, to distinguish genuine missing values from coding omissions.

It is usually better to record date of birth (which is fixed) rather than age which depends on the date of the questionnaire. However, it is better to record actual age than simply age group, because it is easy for a computer to group age in whatever way the investigator requires at the time of analysis. There are many ways in which questions can lead to biased responses. For example it is usually better to ask directly 'how much alcohol do you drink?' and give the subject the option of replying 'none' than to first ask 'do you drink alcohol?', which has an implicit judgement in it. Questions of the 'when did you stop beating your wife' variety can lead to a large number of missing answers. There are many other examples of how questions should be coded to facilitate the analysis and make it easier for the responder; many of these are discussed by Moser and Kalton (1971) among others.

(c) Choice of sample and of control subjects

The question of whether one has a representative sample is a typical problem faced by statisticians. For example, it used to be believed that migraine was associated with intelligence, perhaps on the grounds that people who used their brains were more likely to get headaches. However, a population study by Waters (1971) failed to reveal any social class gradient and, by implication, any association with intelligence. The fallacy arose because intelligent people were more likely to consult their physician about migraine, and so were not representative of the whole population of migraine sufferers. The physicians failed to see the less intelligent migraine sufferers, the less intelligent being less likely to consult with their physicians.

In many studies an investigator will wish to compare patients suffering from a certain disease with healthy (control) subjects. The choice of the appropriate control population is crucial to a correct interpretation of the results. This is discussed further in Chapter 2.

(d) Design of study

It has been emphasised that design deserves as much consideration as analysis, and a statistician can provide advice on design. In a clinical trial, for example, what is known as a double-blind randomised design is nearly always preferable (see Chapter 2) but not always achievable. In some situations patients can act as their own controls; in others this is not possible. It may be impossible to randomise treatments to individuals, but possibly one could randomise so that all patients at a particular centre get the same treatment but the treatment assigned to a particular centre is allocated at random. This device is particularly common if the treatment is an intervention. It might be impossible to prevent individuals knowing which treatment they are receiving but it should be possible to shield their assessors from knowing. Methods of randomisation and design issues are discussed in Chapter 2.

(e) Laboratory experiments

Medical investigators often appreciate the effect that biological variation has in patients, but overlook or underestimate its presence in the laboratory. In dose–response studies, for example, it is important to assign treatment at random, whether the experimental units are humans, animals or test-tubes. A statistician can also advise on quality control of routine laboratory measurements and the measurement of within- and between-observer variation. Techniques such as bioassay have been developed in collaboration with statisticians. Problems in comparing one method of making a measurement with another can also be usefully approached using statistical methods.

(f) Displaying data

A well-chosen figure can summarise the results of a study very concisely. A statistician can help by advising on the best methods of displaying data. For example, when plotting histograms, choice of the group interval can affect the shape of the plotted distribution; with too wide an interval important features of the data will be obscured; too narrow an interval and random variation in the data may distract attention from the shape of the underlying distribution. Advice on displaying data is given in Chapter 4.

(g) Choice of summary statistics and statistical analysis

The summary statistics used and the analysis undertaken must reflect the design of the study and the nature of the data. In some situations, for example, a median is a better measure of location than a mean. In a matched study, it is important to produce an estimate of the difference between matched pairs, and an estimate of the reliability of that difference. For example, in a study to examine blood pressure measured in a seated patient compared with that measured when the patient is lying down, it is insufficient simply to report statistics for seated and lying patients separately. The important statistic is the change in blood pressure as the patient changes position and it is the mean and variability of this statistic that we are interested in. This is further discussed in Chapter 10.

Any analysis must take into account potential confounding factors that might account for the observed result. A statistician can advise on the choice of summary statistics, the type of analysis and the presentation of the results.

1.5 FURTHER READING

An excellent introductory text, which concentrates mainly on analysis of studies, but also covers aspects of design, is Bland (1987). A much lengthier and more detailed account is given by Armitage and Berry (1987). Colton (1974), and Bourke, Daly and McGilvray (1985) are intermediate texts. These texts contain far more detail on analysis than would be necessary for an appreciation of statistical usage as presented in the medical journals. Pocock (1983) is a very useful book for the design and analysis of clinical trials, as is Strike (1981) for the analysis of laboratory data. Lindley and Scott (1984) provide statistical tables for looking up exact probabilities and Machin and Campbell (1987) provide tables for computing sample sizes for medical studies.

Chapter 2

Design

Summary

This chapter emphasises the importance, when planning a study, of defining clearly the objectives of the study, the preference for clinically important questions and the choice of a particular design.

The major distinguishing features of different designs are described, that is whether they are longitudinal or cross-sectional, prospective or retrospective, deliberate intervention or observational, randomised or non-randomised. If the subjects are paired or matched in some way, then the analysis should take this into account. The importance of randomised studies is stressed and details of how randomisation can be effected are also described.

2.1 INTRODUCTION

The purpose of this chapter is to review different types of design of study, and to outline the strengths and weaknesses of different designs. Considerable effort at the planning stage of a study can avoid potential pitfalls in the conduct of the study and give a clear guide to a satisfactory analysis and summary.

2.2 DEFINING THE OBJECTIVES

Table 2.1 summarises the first points to consider when one is planning a study or reading a study report.

Thus before conducting a clinical study of any kind one must first specify the questions to be answered. In most situations it is difficult to identify a single question. For example, if one were asked to investigate the efficacy of a new drug, one question is: 'Is the new drug better than the current medication used for this condition?' A second question may

7

Table 2.1   Planning a study – determining the objectives

(1)   What is the major objective of the study?
(2)   Is it unambiguously defined?
(3)   Is it clinically worth while?
(4)   Are secondary objectives clearly stated?

concern the detection (if any) of undesirable side-effects and there may be additional subsidiary yet important questions. However, it is always desirable to have a principal objective in view. Secondary objectives should be clearly defined as such and should be as few as possible. One must also consider whether the basic question is worth answering. For example, if a test drug is only a very minor modification of the standard, any difference in efficacy is likely to be small and hence may have no *clinical significance*. A trial of the new drug may indicate that the new drug is *statistically significantly* superior to the standard drug, albeit by only a very small amount. Such a result is unlikely to change clinical practice. Questions that have already been posed and the answers to which are clear from the medical literature, are best avoided.

At an early stage one must define appropriate endpoints. For example, in the trial of a new drug, it is necessary to define efficacy unambiguously, and in such a way that it can be verified easily in each patient with the condition under treatment.

A medical study requires careful planning as well as execution and it is usually worth while to put the design in a formal protocol. In the protocol it is necessary to define all aspects of the study from design to an indication of the form of the final analysis. The protocol then provides the reference document as the study progresses. More specific details concerned with the contents of a protocol are described in Section 8.3.

It should be emphasised that the form of the statistical analysis is determined by the type of study design used.

In many situations it is important to separate research activities from day-to-day clinical practice. For example, it may not be usual practice in a busy clinic to record a patient's blood pressure very carefully nor to ensure the necessary rest time before the blood pressure is measured, since the purpose of measurement is simply to decide if the patient is or is not obviously hypertensive. However, if the patient was in a clinical trial to determine changes in blood pressure induced by treatment, more care is required in both standardisation of measurement techniques and level of detail in recording the measurement. For clinical studies it is usually worth having special data forms which prompt the investigator to obtain all the appropriate information whether it be in the laboratory, clinic or hospital ward.

2.3 TYPES OF STUDY

The classification of a research report into study type before detailed reading is often useful. It can alert the reader to critical issues that may be unfamiliar to them, and can guide them to the appropriate analysis. A report that is difficult to classify may have failed to communicate clearly aspects of the design of the study that are crucial for a proper understanding and evaluation. Bailar and Mosteller (1986) describe a classification of biomedical research, and this is summarised in Table 2.2.

Table 2.2   A classification of biomedical research reports

I.   *Longitudinal studies*
A.   Prospective studies
(1)   Deliberate interventions
(a)   randomised
(b)   non-randomised
(2)   Observational studies
B.   Retrospective studies
(1)   Deliberate intervention
(2)   Observational studies
II.   *Cross-sectional studies*
A.   Disease description
B.   Diagnosis and staging
(1)   Abnormal ranges
(2)   Disease severity
C.   Disease processes

Source: Bailer and Mosteller (1986).

The major division is between longitudinal and cross-sectional studies. A longitudinal study investigates a process over time; examples might be a clinical trial, a cohort study or a case-control study. Cross-sectional studies describe a phenomenon fixed in time; an example might be a description of the TNM staging system for breast cancer. Most studies of the effect of external factors on human beings would tend to be longitudinal, whereas laboratory studies of biological processes are often cross-sectional. Longitudinal studies are divided into prospective and retrospective studies. In prospective studies subjects are grouped according to 'exposure' to some factor. Thus the total period of use of a particular oral contraceptive by a woman could be the exposure, and the outcome of interest, prospectively observed, may be the development or otherwise of breast cancer in that woman. In retrospective studies, subjects are first divided by the outcome, such as women with breast cancer (the cases) and women who do not have breast cancer (the controls). The 'exposure' effect such as the period of use of the oral contraceptive is then determined retrospectively.

2.4 THE RANDOMISED CLINICAL TRIAL

(a) Randomisation

A clinical trial is defined as a prospective study comparing the efficacy of a test treatment or intervention against a control treatment in human subjects. Randomisation is a procedure in which the play of chance enters into the assignment of a subject to test or control, so that the assignment cannot be predicted in advance. The main point is that randomisation tends to produce study groups comparable in *unknown* as well as known factors likely to influence the outcome apart from the actual treatment being given itself. Randomisation also guarantees that statistical tests will have valid significance levels, although this is a rather technical point. The need for randomisation is often not appreciated and it is important to distinguish it from *haphazard* allocation. A typical haphazard allocation method is where the patients are assigned to test or control treatment alternately as they enter the clinic. The investigator might argue that the factors that determine precisely which subject enters the clinic at a given time are random and hence treatment allocation is also random. The problem here is that it is possible to predict which treatment the patients will receive as soon as or even before they are screened for eligibility for the trial. This knowledge may then influence the investigator when determining which patients are admitted to the trial and which patients are not. This in turn may lead to bias in the final treatment comparisons. Methods of randomisation are described in Section 2.13.

(b) Parallel designs

In a parallel design, one group receives the test treatment, and one group the control. This is represented in Figure 2.1.

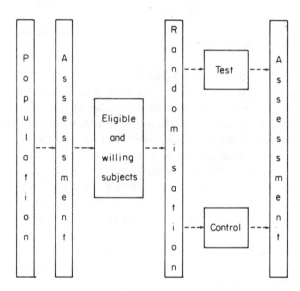

Figure 2.1   A parallel design clinical trial

Example from the literature

Thomas (1987) randomly allocated patients who consulted him for minor illnesses to either a 'positive' or a 'negative' consultation. After two weeks he found that 64% of those receiving a positive consultation got better compared with only 39% of those who received a negative consultation.

Statistical analysis was used to show that these differences were unlikely to have arisen by chance. The conclusion was therefore that a patient who received a positive consultation was more likely to get better.

(c) Cross-over designs

In a cross-over design the subjects receive both the test and the control treatments in a randomised order.

Example from the literature

Scott, Knowles and Beaver (1984) conducted a trial of Acarbose or placebo in non-insulin-dependent diabetics. After a two-week run-in period to allow patients to become familiar with details of the trial, 18 patients were allocated by random draw to either active or placebo tablets. After one month individuals were crossed over to the alternative tablet, for a further month. In the final week of each of the one-month treatment periods the percentage glycosolated haemoglobin (HbA1%) was measured.

The two period cross-over design is described in Figure 2.2. The difference between HbA1% levels after placebo and Acarbose was calculated for each patient. The average difference between levels after active and placebo treatments of 0.3%, with standard deviation of 0.5%, indicated that Acarbose had little effect on HbA1%.

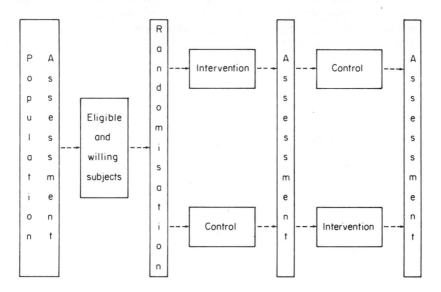

Figure 2.2   A two-period cross-over design clinical trial

One difficulty with cross-over designs is the possibility that the effect of the particular treatment use in the first period will carry over to the second period. This may then interfere with how the treatment scheduled for the second period will act, and thus affect the final comparison between the two treatments (the carry-over effect). To allow for this possibility, a *washout* period, in which no treatment is given, should be included between successive treatment periods.

A cross-over study results in a paired (or matched) analysis. It is incorrect to analyse the trial ignoring this pairing.

Sampson and Prescott (1981) suggest a design to compare two treatments in four periods. Such a design allows for estimation of both the treatment and the carry-over effects.

Further issues in the design and analysis of randomised clinical trials will be discussed in Chapter 8.

2.5 NON-RANDOMISED STUDIES

(a) Historical controls

In the discussion related to clinical trials the need for randomised allocation of treatments was indicated. In certain circumstances, however, randomisation is not possible; one good example is any study involving heart transplantation and subsequent survival experience of the patients. It would be difficult to imagine randomising between heart transplantation and some other alternative, and so the best one can do in such circumstances is to compare survival time following transplant with previous patients suffering from the same condition when transplants were not available. Such patients are termed *historical controls*. A second possibility is to make comparisons with those in which a donor did not become available before patient death. There are difficulties with either approach. One is that those with the most serious problems will die more quickly. The presence of any waiting time for a suitable donor implies that only the less critical will survive this waiting time. This can clearly bias comparisons of survival experience in the transplanted and non-transplanted groups.

Example from the literature

Campbell, Browne and Waters (1985) evaluated a health promotion campaign by a general practitioner. Questionnaires asking about amount of exercise taken were sent to random samples of subjects before and after the campaign, both in the village where the practitioner worked and in a control village which had no campaign exposure.

In the 'intervention' village, the percentage of people who exercised until breathless more than once a week changed from 39% to 51%. However, in the control village the change was from 38% to 45%. The conclusion was that there had been a general increase in the amount of exercise taken, possibly due to general publicity received by both villages, and that the effect of the general practitioner, if present, was at most minor. In this example it is clear that the design of the study precluded randomisation of individuals to the campaign or control village.

(b) Pre-test–post-test studies

A *pre-test–post-test* study is one in which a group of individuals are measured, then subjected to a treatment or intervention, and then measured again. The purpose of the study is to measure the effect of treatment. The major problem is ascribing the change in the measurement to the treatment since other factors may also have changed in that interval.

Example from the literature

Christie (1979) describes an example where a before-and-after comparison is misleading. He describes a consecutive series of patients admitted to hospital with stroke in 1974 who were then followed prospectively until death and their survival time calculated. In

1978 the study was repeated so that a computed tomography (CT) head scanner which had been installed in the intervening period could be evaluated.

Successive patients in the 1978 series who had had a CT scan were matched by age, diagnosis and level of consciousness with patients in the 1974 series. Outcome was measured by length of survival from onset of disease. The results, given in Table 2.3, appeared to show a marked improvement in the 1978 patients over those from 1974. This was presumed to be due to the CT scanner. However, the study was extended to an analysis of the 1978 patients who had not had a CT scan compared with a matched group in 1974 using identical matching criteria. The formal statistical analysis found a very similar result with a significant improvement in 1978. Thus, whether or not patients had received a CT scan, the treatment had improved over the years.

Table 2.3   Example of a misleading before-and-after study

	CT scan in 1978	No CT scan in 1978
Pairs with identical outcomes 1974 and 1978	18	38
Pairs where 1978 better than 1974	9	34
Pairs where 1978 worse than 1974	2	17
Total	29	89
p-value	0.02	0.006

Source: Christie (1979).

The explanation of the apparent anomaly is that other improvements had occurred between 1974 and 1978. In the absence of the control study, with no CT scan, the investigators may well have concluded that the installation of a CT head scanner had improved patient survival time.

However in certain circumstances before-and-after studies without control groups are unavoidable.

Example from the literature

Mills, Campbell and Waters (1986) evaluated whether a British Government education campaign had increased the level of public knowledge of AIDS. Questionnaires were sent to random samples of the electoral roll of Southampton before and after a newspaper advertisement campaign.

The investigators found, for example, that 33% of the population knew what the initials AIDS stood for before the campaign, and only 34% after the campaign. They concluded that the campaign appeared to have had little effect on the level of knowledge of AIDS in the general population.

Since the Government campaign covered the whole country, no realistic control group was possible.

2.6 COHORT STUDIES

(a) Design

A *cohort* is a component of a population identified so that its characteristics, for example, causes of death or numbers contracting a certain disease, can be ascertained as it ages through time.

The term 'cohort' is often used to describe those born during a particular year but can be extended to describe any designated group of persons who are traced over a period of time. Thus, for example, we may refer to a cohort born in 1900, or to a cohort of people who ever worked in a particular factory. A *cohort study*, which may also be referred to as a follow-up, longitudinal or prospective study, is one in which subsets of a defined population can be identified who have been exposed (or will be exposed) to a factor which may influence the probability of occurrence of a given disease or other outcome. A study may follow two groups of subjects, one group exposed to a potential toxic hazard, the other not, to see if the exposure influences, for example, the occurrence of certain types of cancers. Cohort studies are usually confined to studies determining and investigating aetiological factors, and do not allocate the equivalent of treatments.

The design and progress of a cohort study are shown in Figure 2.3.

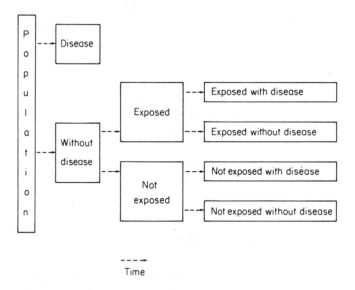

Figure 2.3   Progress of a cohort study

The interpretation of cohort studies is often more difficult than that of a randomised trial as bias may influence the measure of interest. For example, to determine in a cohort study if the rate of cardiovascular disease is raised in men sterilised by vasectomy it is necessary to have a comparison group of non-vasectomised men. However, comparisons between these two groups of men may be biased as it is clearly not possible to randomise men to sterilisation or non-sterilisation groups. Men who are seeking sterilisation would certainly not accept the 'no sterilisation' option. Thus the comparison that will be made here is between those men who opt for sterilisation against those who do not and there may be inherent biases present when comparisons are made between the two groups. For example, the vasectomised men may be fitter or better educated than the non-vasectomised men and this may influence cardiovascular disease rates.

In the design of a cohort study, careful consideration before commencement of the study must be taken to identify and subsequently measure important prognostic variables that may differ between the exposure groups. Provided they are recorded, differences in these baseline characteristics between groups can be adjusted for in the final analysis.

Example from the literature

Schatzkin *et al.* (1987) studied 7188 women aged 25 to 74 who were examined from 1971 to 1975 as part of the National Health and Nutrition Examination Survey (NHANES 1) in the USA. Questions about alcohol consumption were included. The subjects were traced between 1981 and 1984 and cases of breast cancer identified.

The investigators found that for drinkers the risk of breast cancer was 50% higher than for non-drinkers. Even allowing for other risk factors such as menopausal status, obesity and smoking, the investigators were able to establish a link between alcohol consumption and subsequent incidence of breast cancer.

In this case the principal use of statistical analysis is to try and sort out whether it is really alcohol consumption that is causing the increased breast cancer incidence, or if it is due to one of the large number of other factors that are associated with alcohol consumption.

Example from the literature

Campbell, Elwood, Mckean and Waters (1985) studied 1438 women aged 45–74 who were examined in 1967 and their haemoglobin levels determined. They were then followed up for mortality in 1979. The proportion followed-up was 99%.

The investigators found that the mean level of haemoglobin at the time of the first survey in women who subsequently died of cancer was 12.3 g/dl compared with 12.8 g/dl in those who were still alive at follow-up. The authors were able to establish that the relationship between haemoglobin and cancer was unlikely to have arisen by chance, and could not be explained by other known risk factors such as smoking habit.

(b) Size of study

The required size of a cohort study depends not only on the size of the risk being investigated but also on the incidence of the particular condition under investigation. In the vasectomy example, cardiovascular events are not particularly rare among a cohort of men aged 40–50 and this may determine that the cohort of middle-aged men be investigated. On the other hand, if a rare condition were being investigated very few events would be observed perhaps in many thousands of subjects whether exposed to the 'insult' of interest or not. This usually prevents the use of cohort studies to investigate aetiological factors in rare diseases.

(c) Problems in interpretation

When the cohort is made up of employed as opposed to unemployed individuals, the risk of dying in the first few years of follow-up is generally less than that of the general population. This is known as the 'healthy worker' effect. It is due to the fact that people who are sick are less likely to be employed. It is also known that people who respond to questionnaires are likely to be fitter than those who do not. Both can lead to problems in the interpretation of risks from employed populations. Another problem arises when follow-up is poor, or when it is better for the exposed group than for the unexposed group. Are the people lost to follow-up different in any way and could a poor follow-up bias the conclusions?

d) Post-marketing surveillence

Post-marketing surveillance is a particular type of cohort study carried out on a population of people receiving a new drug. In such an example, a drug that is in routine use nationwide may be monitored – not for its efficacy but for any untoward medical event happening to patients receiving the drug. The incidence of such adverse events with the new drug is then compared with the incidence in patients receiving alternatives to the new medicine.

2.7 CASE-CONTROL STUDIES

(a) Design

A case-control study, also known as a case-referent study or retrospective study, starts with the identification of persons with the disease (or other outcome variable) of interest, and a suitable control (reference) group of persons without the disease. The relationship of a risk factor to the disease is examined by comparing the diseased and non-diseased with regard to how frequently the risk factor is present. If the variable under consideration is quantitative, the average levels of the risk factor in the cases and controls are utilised.

The design and progress of a case-control study are shown in Figure 2.4.

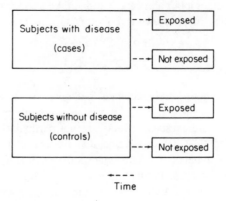

Figure 2.4   Progress of a case-control study

There are two possible variations in design. The control subjects can be chosen to match individual cases for certain important variables leading to what is known as a matched design. In many circumstances the matching criteria may include age and sex. However, it is a common misconception that there must be matching criteria in all case-control studies. Alternatively the controls can be a sample from a suitable non-diseased population, leading to an unmatched design. The statistical analysis will reflect the chosen design.

(b) Unmatched study

Example from the literature

Olsen, Petring and Rossing (1987) studied 7 women with primary Raynaud's phenomenon and 10 healthy women, and also 7 men with vibration white finger and 8 healthy men. The controls were medical students. They compared the vasoconstrictor response to sitting between the cases and controls.

The authors used statistics to summarise the data and to show that the augmented response in the cases compared with the controls could not have arisen by chance. A major consideration here is whether the difference between cases and controls is due to the disease in the cases, or whether other factors could explain it. Does the fact that medical students are likely to be younger and healthier than the typical members of the diseased population explain the size of difference observed?

(c) Selection of controls

The general principle in selecting controls is to choose subjects who might have been cases in the study (Rothman, 1986), and to select them independently of the exposure variable. Thus if the cases were all treated in one particular hospital the controls should represent people who, had they developed the disease , would also have gone to the same hospital. Note that this is not the same as selecting hospital controls (see the example below). It is incorrect to require the controls to be representative of all those subjects without the disease, as has been suggested in some textbooks. It is also not correct to require that the control group are alike in every respect to the cases, apart from not having the disease of interest. An example of this 'over-matching' is given by Horwitz and Feinstein (1978) in a study of oestrogens and endometrial cancer. The cases and controls were both drawn from women who had been evaluated by uterine dilatation and curettage. Such a control group is inappropriate because agents that cause one disease in an organ often cause other diseases or symptoms in that organ. In this case it is possible that oestrogens cause other diseases of the endometrium, which requires the women to have dilatation and so present as possible controls.

The choice of the appropriate control population is crucial to a correct interpretation of the results. A typical problem when the cases are patients admitted to hospital is whether to choose hospital or population controls.

Example from the literature

In a study of the role of familial environment in the development of mental illness in children by Oleinick *et al.* (1966) two controls were selected for each case seen at a psychiatric clinic. One was a *hospital* control, a child who had had an appendectomy or tonsillectomy and hence attended a paediatric clinic. The other was a *population* control drawn from the local community.

The investigators studied aetiological factors such as the disruption of the parents' marital relationship, and found that the strength of the association with mental illness for the hospital controls was between that for the cases and that for the population controls. This implies that the hospital controls had certain characteristics that rendered them closer to the mental illness cases than was the case for the population controls.

(d) Confounding

Confounding arises when the effects of two processes are not separated. In such cases the apparent effect of an exposure on risk can be distorted by other factors that also influence the outcome. Confounding has also been termed 'Simpson's paradox' and can most easily be illustrated by means of a numerical example. Consider a situation in which a disease is related to two possible exposures A and B. The results are given in Table 2.4.

In Table 2.4(a) it would appear clear that exposure to A increases the risk of disease. However, when the same data are split by exposure to B in Table 2.4(b), it appears that exposure to A is in fact *protective* of disease. Factor B is termed the *confounding* factor. To be a confounder a factor must be both related to the exposure of interest, and have a real effect on the disease process. This is clearly the case in Table 2.4, since the disease is more prevalent when B is present (80/100 compared with 6/100 when it is not), and one is more likely to have been exposed to A if one has been exposed to B. As an example, it has been reported in several studies that asthmatics appear to be at lower risk of cancer than non-asthmatics. However, asthmatics are also less likely to smoke, and non-smokers are less likely to contract cancer than smokers, so smoking is a confounding factor in this case. In such a case it would be more appropriate to restrict the study to non-smoking asthmatic cases and non-smoking controls.

Table 2.4   An example of confounding or 'Simpson's Paradox'

(a) Disease	Exposure to A	
	Yes	No
Present	64	22
Absent	66	48
	130	70
Percentage with the disease	49%	31%

(b)	Exposure to B		No exposure to B	
	Exposure to A		Exposure to A	
Disease	Yes	No	Yes	No
Present	63	17	1	5
Absent	17	3	49	45
	80	20	50	50
Percentage with the disease	79%	85%	2%	10%

(e) Matched study

The main purpose of *matching* is to permit the use of efficient analytical methods to control for confounding variables that might influence the case-control comparison. In addition it can lead to a clear identification of appropriate controls. However, matching can be wasteful and costly if the matching criteria lead to many available controls being discarded because they fail the matching criteria. In fact if controls are too closely matched to their respective cases, the relative risk (see Chapter 9) may be underestimated. Usually it is only worth while matching on at most two or three variables which are presumed or known to influence outcome, common variables being age, sex and social class in certain types of epidemiological studies.

Example from the literature

Brown, Pottern and Hoover (1987) studied all cases of testicular cancer in a defined area from 1 January 1976 to 30 June 1986. The controls were men in the same hospital as the cases, who were within 2 years of age and belonged to the same ethnic group as the cases but suffering from a malignancy other than testicular cancer.

From the study the investigators concluded that those with undescended testes at birth had a higher risk of developing testicular cancer.

(f) Limitations of case-control studies

Ascertainment of exposure in case-control studies relies on previously recorded data or on memory, and it is difficult to ensure lack of bias between the cases and the controls. Since they are suffering a disease, cases are likely to be more motivated to recall possible risk factors. One of the major difficulties with case-control studies is in the selection of a suitable control group, and this has often been a major source of criticism of published case-control studies.

2.8 CROSS-SECTIONAL SURVEYS

Suppose an investigator wishes to determine the prevalence of menstrual flushing in women in the ages 45–60 (see Smith and Waters, 1983). Then an appropriate design may be a survey of women in that age group by means of a postal questionnaire. In such a situation, this type of survey may be conducted at, for example, a town, county or national level. However a prerequisite before such a survey is conducted is a list of women in the corresponding age groups. Once such a list is obtained it may be possible to send a postal questionnaire to all women on the list. More usually one may wish to draw a sample from the list. The sampling proportion will have to be chosen carefully, and the questionnaire be sent to this sample. It is important that the selection is made by an appropriate randomisation technique as described in Section 2.13(d).

   In some situations a visit by an interviewer to those included in the sample may be more appropriate. However, this may be costly both in time and money and will require the training of personnel. As a consequence this will usually involve a smaller sample than that possible by means of a postal questionnaire. On the other hand, response rates to questionnaires may be low; for example, Smith and Waters (1983) quote a 68%

response. A low response rate can cause considerable difficulty in interpretation of the results as it can always be argued (whether true or not) that non-responders are atypical with respect to the problem being investigated and therefore estimates of prevalence, necessarily obtained from the responders only, will be inherently biased. Thus in a well designed survey, every attempt should be made to keep the numbers of non-responders to a minimum. The potential response rate is taken into account when estimating sample size.

Volunteers often present considerable problems in cross-sectional surveys. When the object of interest is a relationship within subjects, for example physiological responses to increasing doses of a drug, then one cannot avoid the use of volunteers. However, suppose a survey was to be carried out on the prevalence of hypertension in the community. One approach would be to ask volunteers to come forward by advertising in the local newspaper. The difficulty here is that people may volunteer simply because they are worried about their blood pressure, and there is no way one can ascertain the response rate, or investigate reasons why people did not volunteer. A better approach would be to take a random sample from the community, either from an electoral roll, general practioners' lists or a telephone list and then invite each one individually to have their blood pressure measured. In that way the response rate is known and the non-responders identified.

Market research organisations have complex sampling schemes that often contain elements of randomisation. However, in essence they are *grab* or *convenience* samples, in that only subjects who are available to the interviewer can be questioned. So-called *quota* samples ensure that the sample is representative of the general population in say, age, sex and social class structure. The problems in the interpretation of quota samples are discussed in detail by Moser and Kalton (1971). They are not recommended for use in medical research.

It is usually good practice to make any questionnaire, whether self-completed by the recipient or by an interviewer, as short and as clearly worded as possible. Some compromise must be reached between the desirable length and complexity of a questionnaire and extracting all the information from the subject which may influence, in the example considered above, the prevalence of menstrual flushes. The questionnaire itself needs to be validated, perhaps in a small pilot study. Some types of survey may not require response from the individuals themselves. An example would be a case-note or databank survey of patients with a particular condition, perhaps patients with diabetes, in which the investigator may be interested in what factors determine whether or not the patients develop retinopathy. Case-note studies are often unsatisfactory as the notes are not usually collected for research purposes and critical 'research' items may not be recorded.

Compared with cohort studies a number of biases are possible in cross-sectional studies. Consider a cross-sectional study that reveals a negative association between height and age. Possible interpretations include: people shrink as they get older, younger generations are getting taller, or tall people have a higher mortality than short people!

One of the differences between a cohort study, a case-control study and a cross-sectional study is that in the latter subjects are included without reference to either their exposure or their disease. Cross-sectional studies usually deal with exposures that do not change, such as blood type or chronic smoking habit. However, in occupational studies a cross-sectional study might contain all workers in a factory, and their exposures determined by a retrospective work-history. A cross-sectional study resembles a case-control study except that the numbers of cases are not known in advance, but are simply the cases present at the time of the survey.

Example from the literature

Wynne *et al*. (1987) studied the effectiveness of basic life-support skills in 53 nurses attending a course. One aim of the study was to examine the relationship between self-assessed and actual skills.

The use of statistics comes in deciding whether any relationship found between self-assessed and actual skills could have arisen by chance. Wynne *et al*. also found that 30 of the nurses were completely ineffective at life-support skills, a level comparable to that reported in the USA. The investigators interviewed all nurses attending a training course; however, the use of their results by others requires an assumption that the group of nurses studied is in some way representative or typical of other groups of nurses.

2.9 REFERENCE RANGES

A common problem in for example clinical chemistry is to determine reference ranges for a particular test. Once the reference range is determined, any patient with a suspected pathology may have the test and the result compared with the reference range. A result outside the reference range may then be taken as confirmation of the pathology.

In determining reference ranges it is necessary to first test the method on subjects without the underlying pathology under consideration. For this purpose 'normal healthy volunteers' are utilised. These are often chosen to be cooperative colleagues in the investigators' laboratory or medical students anxious to learn. Such groups may not in fact constitute an appropriate 'normal' group in every instance. For example, workers in one laboratory are exposed to a similar working environment which may influence their blood biochemistry in a way not experienced by others and hence their use may lead to inappropriate reference ranges. It follows that volunteers should be selected so as to exclude possible biases. We return to such problems later.

Example from the literature

Sherry *et al*. (1988) collected blood samples from 76 healthy, afebrile children, ranging in age from 2 to 36 months, and determined the serum prealbumin concentration. All the children had been hospitalised with viral meningitis for up to 10 days in a period one to two months before the study.

The authors stated, with little evidence presented, that the prealbumin levels were representative of those for normal children. They quoted the normal range as 2 standard deviations (see Appendix A2) either side of the mean. The results gave a normal range of 116 to 282 mg/l.

The main use of statistics in this case is in the selection of a range so that in future samples of normal children, a fixed proportion will fall outside the range. The limits are usually chosen so that 5% of apparently 'normal' children will fall outside the range.

The use of 2 standard deviations either side of the mean implies that the authors have assumed a particular distribution for serum prealbumin concentration. Confusingly this is usually referred to as the Normal (see Section 5.2) distribution. The statistical problems associated with the calculation of normal ranges have been discussed by Tango (1986). Further discussion of the interpretation of laboratory results has been given by Fraser and Fogarty (1989).

2.10 METHOD COMPARISON STUDIES

Another feature of laboratory work is the evaluation of new instruments. It is usual in such studies to compare results obtained from the new with that obtained from some standard. Alternatively, two devices may be proposed for measuring the same quantity and one may wish to determine which is the better.

Example from the literature

Belsey, Goitein and Baer (1987) compared the results from a table-top chemistry analyser with those obtained from standard laboratory techniques.

They found that for 6 out of 7 assays, the error of the machine was well within the allowable analytical error ranges around the relevant medical decision level. They concluded that the table-top analyser was acceptably accurate and precise using correlations with several reference measurements as the determining criteria.

Bland and Altman (1986) provide useful guidelines for assessing agreement between two methods of clinical measurement. In particular they argue against the use of the correlation coefficient (see Chapter 10) as was used by the authors in the above example.

2.11 STUDIES OF DIAGNOSTIC TESTS

Diagnostic tests have three main uses: diagnosis of disease, screening and patient management.

(a) Diagnosis of disease

In the process of making a diagnosis for a particular patient, a clinician establishes a set of diagnostic alternatives or hypotheses. He then attempts to reduce these by progressively ruling out specific diseases. He will require tests both to exclude certain diagnoses and tests to confirm certain diagnoses. Given a particular diagnosis, a good test should indicate either that the disease is unlikely or that it is probable.

(b) Screening

The main purpose in screening asymptomatic patients is to detect diseases whose morbidity and mortality can be reduced by early detection and treatment. A number of points need to be clarified before screening should be considered:

 (i) The disease in question should be common enough to justify the effort to detect it. If the disease is very rare, then the number of lives saved by screening is going to be small.
 (ii) The disease should be accompanied by significant morbidity if not treated.
 (iii) Effective therapy must exist to alter its natural history.
 (iv) Detection and treatment of the presymptomatic state should result in benefits beyond those obtained through treatment of the early symptomatic patient.

(c) Patient management

When patients have an established disease, tests are used to monitor progress of the disease, to aid prognosis and to evaluate the effects of treatment.

Example from the literature

Campbell *et al.* (1989) conducted a survey of acute lower respiratory tract infection in a community in Africa. They found that a fever greater than 38.5 °C or a respiratory rate greater than 60 breaths/min were the most accurate clinical signs of infection.

These results differed from those found in hospital-based studies. They claimed that the case fatality rates would be reduced if primary health-care workers could identify the most serious forms of lower respiratory tract infection and then deal with them appropriately. The use of statistics comes in the selection of subjects, the identification of the correct measures of accuracy, and the choice of the best of these.

   Diagnostic tests are discussed in more detail in Chapter 3.

2.12 MORE COMPLEX DESIGNS

(a) Factorial designs

Example from the literature

McMaster, Nichols and Machin (1985) describe a study to evaluate breast self-examination teaching materials. Four different experimental conditions were evaluated in health centre waiting rooms in which women were waiting to see their general practitioner. These were:

A No leaflets or tape–slide programme available (control)
B Leaflets displayed
C Tape–slide programme
D Leaflets displayed and tape–slide programme

The evaluation of the four experimental conditions was conducted on four weekdays (Monday to Thursday) for four weeks. In order to eliminate bias, a Latin square experimental procedure was employed, such that each experimental condition was evaluated on each of the four weekdays.

The use of this 2×2 factorial design enabled two questions to be asked simultaneously. Groups A and B versus C and D measured the value of the tape–slide programme while groups A and C versus B and D measured the value of the leaflets.

(b) Dose–response studies

An important type of investigation is one which studies dose–response relationships. In these cases the dose is under the control of the investigator.

Example from the literature

Beasley, Rafferty and Holgate (1987) describe an experiment in which patients are given progressively increasing doses of a bronchoconstrictor and their lung fuction measured at each dose.

The outcome measure may be the slope of the dose–response curve, or the dose which achieves a given response such as the PD_{20} which is the dose required to reduce lung fuction to 20% of baseline. The dose response can be estimated using *regression* techniques (described in Chapter 7). Choice of appropriate doses is important for efficient estimation of the dose–response relation. For example, it would be sensible to concentrate doses around the expected PD_{20} point to get an efficient estimate of it.

(c) Mixed studies

Any study may consist of various features of the basic designs outlined in Table 2.2. For example, a clinical trial comparing two treatments is longitudinal in nature (similar to a cohort study), it may involve laboratory investigations of subgroups of patients, and of course each patient represents a *single case design* in that the protocol treatment schedule may depend on the patient's response at various stages during a trial. In a cohort study, prognostic factors may be evaluated retrospectively, and the results then analysed as if the design were a case-control one. In some circumstances in can be difficult to find a single label to cover all aspects of a particular study.

2.13 METHODS OF RANDOMISATION

(a) Simple randomisation

The simplest randomisation device is a coin which if tossed will land with a particular face upwards with probability one-half. Thus one way to assign treatments of patients at random in a clinical trial would be to assign treatment A whenever a particular side of the coin turned up, and B when the obverse arises. An alternative might be to roll a six-sided die: if an even number falls A is given, if an odd number, B. Such procedures are termed *simple randomisation*. It is usual to generate the randomisation list in advance of recruiting the first patient. This has several advantages: it removes the possibility of the physician not randomising properly, it will usually be more efficient in that a list may be computer generated very quickly, and it allows some difficulties with simple randomisation to be avoided.

To avoid the use of a die for simple randomisation one can produce a table of random numbers such as Table T4. Although Table T4 is in fact computer generated, the table is similar to that which would result from throwing a ten-sided die, with faces marked 0 to 9, on successive occasions. The digits are grouped into blocks merely for ease of reading. The table is used by first choosing a point of entry, perhaps with a pin, and deciding the direction of movement, for example along the rows or down the columns. Suppose the pin chooses the entry in the 10th row and 13th column of Table T4 and it had been decided to move along the rows; the first 10 digits then give 534 55425 67; even numbers assigned to A and odd to B then generate BBA BBAAB AB. Thus of the first 10 patients recruited 4 will receive A and 6 B.

Although simple randomisation gives equal probability for each patient to receive A or B it does not ensure, as indeed was the case with our example, that at the end of patient recruitment to the trial equal numbers of patients received A and B. In fact even in relatively large trials the discrepancy from the desired equal numbers of patients per treatment can be quite large. In small trials the discrepancy can be very serious, perhaps resulting in too few patients in one group to give acceptable statistical precision of the corresponding treatment efficacy.

(b) Blocked randomisation

To avoid such a problem balanced or restricted randomisation techniques are used. In this case the allocation procedure is organised in such a way that equal numbers are allocated to A and B for every block of a certain number of patients. One method of doing this, say for successive blocks of four patients, is to generate all possible combinations but ignoring those with unequal allocation. The combinations are:

1	AABB	4	BABA
2	ABAB	5	BAAB
3	ABBA	6	BBAA

These combinations are allocated the numbers 1 to 6 and the randomisation table used to generate a sequence of digits. Suppose this sequence was 534 55425 67 as before, then reading from left to right we generate the allocation BAAB ABBA BABA BAAB for the first 16 patients. Such a device ensures that for every four successive patients recruited, balance between A and B is maintained. Should a 0, 7, 8 or 9 occur in the random sequence then these are ignored as there is no associated treatment combination in these cases. It is important that the investigating physician is not aware of the block size, otherwise he or she will come to know, as each block of patients nears completion, the next treatment to be allocated. This knowledge can introduce bias into the allocation process. Such a difficulty can be avoided by changing the block size as recruitment continues.

In trials which involve recruitment in several centres, it is usual to use a stratified randomisation procedure to ensure balanced treatment allocation within centres. Another important use of stratified randomisation in clinical trials occurs when it is known that a particular patient characteristic may be an important prognostic indicator – perhaps good or bad pathology – then equal allocation of treatments within each prognostic group may be desirable. This ensures that treatment comparisons can be made efficiently, allowing for prognostic factors. Stratified randomisation can be extended to more than one stratum, for example, centre and pathology, but it is not usually desirable to go beyond two strata.

One method that can balance a large number of strata is known as *minimisation*. It is described, for example, in Pocock (1983). One difficulty with the method is that it requires details of all patients previously entered into the trial, before allocation can be made.

(c) Carrying out randomisation

Once the randomised list is made, and it is usually best if this is not done by the investigator determining patient eligibility, how is randomisation carried out? One simple way is to have it kept out of the clinic but with someone who can give the randomisation over the telephone. The physician rings the number, gives the necessary patient details, perhaps confirming the protocol entry criteria, and is told which treatment to give, or perhaps a code number of a drug package, if a double-blind trial. It should be noted that if a placebo or standard drug is to be used in a double-blind trial, it should be packaged in exactly the same way as the active treatment. Once determined, treatment should commence as soon as is practicable.

Another device, which is certainly more common in small-scale studies, is to prepare sequentially numbered sealed envelopes which contain the appropriate treatment. The attending physician only opens the envelope once he or she has decided the patient is eligible for the trial and consent has been obtained. The name of the patient is also written on the card containing the treatment allocation and the card returned to the principal investigator immediately. Any unused envelopes are also return to the principal investigator at the end of the study as a check on the randomisation process.

The above discussion has used the example of a randomised control trial comparing two treatments as this is the simplest situation. The method extends relatively easily to more complex designs, however. For example, in the case of a 2×2 factorial design involving four treatments, the treatments, labelled A, B, C and D, could be allocated the digits 01, 23, 45 and 67 respectively. The random sequence 534 55425 67 would then generate CBCCCCBCDD; thus in the first 10 patients none would receive A, two B, six C and two D. Balanced arrangements to give equal numbers of patients per group can be produced by first generating the treatment combinations for blocks of an appropriate size. Of necessity block size must always be a multiple of the number of treatments under investigation.

(d) Random samples in surveys

In a survey a simple randon sample would be obtained first by numbering all the individual members in the target population, and then computer-generating random numbers from that list. Suppose the population totals 600 subjects, then they are numbered 001 through to 600. The random sequence used before would take the first three subjects as 534, 554 and 256, for example. These subjects are then identified on the list and sent the questionnaire. If the population list is not on computer file or is very large, the process of going backwards and forwards to write down addresses of the sample can be a tedious business. Suppose a list is printed on 1000 pages of 100 subjects per page, and a 1% sample is required, then one way is to choose a number between 1 and 100; from our sequence this would be 53, so take the 53rd member of the population on every page. This is clearly logistically easier than taking a random sample of 1000 from a list of 100 000. A 0.5% sample would take someone from every second page but first entry is chosen at random between 001 and 200. Such a device is known as *systematic random sampling*; the choice of starting point is random.

There are other devices which might be appropriate in specific circumstances. For example, for the prevalence of menstrual flushing, rather than sampling the national list containing millions of women, one may first randomly choose from a list of counties, from within each county take a sample of electoral wards, and then obtain only lists for these wards from which to select the women. Such a device is termed *multi-stage random sampling*.

In other circumstances one may wish to ensure that equal numbers of men and women are sampled. Thus the list is divided into strata (men and women) and equal numbers sampled from each stratum.

2.14 POINTS WHEN READING THE LITERATURE

(1) The first step in reading any research report is to decide on the primary objective. See Table 2.1 for the key questions to ask.
(2) Use Table 2.2 and the ensuing discussion to help you decide on the type of study design.
(3) Go to the appropriate chapter of this book to help you decide if the design chosen is an appropriate one, and has been used efficiently. In particular, does the analysis of the study reflect the design (for example has matching been taken into account)?
(4) Pay particular attention to the aspects of randomisation. In a clinical trial, is the method of randomisation described, and if not, could allocation be merely haphazard? In a cross-sectional survey, how were subjects selected? Were they random, or were they 'grab' or 'volunteer' samples?

Chapter 3

Probability and
decision making

Summary

Probability is defined either in terms of the long-term frequency of events, or as a subjective measure of the certainty of an event happening. The ideas associated with the study of probability are illustrated in the context of diagnostic tests. The two major parameters associated with diagnostic tests are the sensitivity and the specificity. The concepts of independent events and mutually exclusive events are discussed, and the use of Bayes' theorem is demonstrated. When the result of a diagnostic test is a continuous variable, there may be difficulty in deciding an appropriate cut-off point and relative operating characteristic (ROC) curves can be used to help with the decision.

3.1 TYPES OF PROBABILITY

We all have an intuitive feel for probability but it is important to distinguish between probabilities applied to single individuals and probabilities applied to groups of individuals. Every year about 600 000 people die in England and Wales. From year to year this number is stable to an extent that surprises some people, and statisticians are able to predict it with better than 99% accuracy. There are about 50 million people in England and Wales and for a single individual, with no information about his age or state of health, the chances of him dying in any particular year are 600 000/50 000 000, or about 12 in 1000. Thus the number of deaths in a particular group can be accurately predicted but it is difficult to predict exactly which individuals in that group are going to die.

The basis of the idea of probability is a sequence of what are known as *independent trials*. To calculate the probability of an individual dying in one year, each one of a group of individuals is given a *trial* over a year and the *event* occurs if the individual dies. The estimate of the probability of dying is the number of deaths divided by the number in the original group. The idea of independence is difficult, but is based on the fact that whether or not one individual survives or dies does not affect the chance of another individual's survival. On a very simple level and where the probability of an event is known in advance, consider tossing one coin 100 times. Each toss of the coin is a 'trial' and the event might be 'heads'. If the coin is unbiased, that is one which has no preference for 'heads' or 'tails', we would expect heads half of the time and thus say the probability of a head is 0.5.

The probability of an event is the proportion of times it occurs in a long sequence of trials. When it is stated that the probability that an unborn child is male is 0.51, the expectation is based on large numbers of previous births. When it is stated that patients with a certain disease have a 50% chance of surviving 5 years, this is based on past experience of other patients with the same disease.

In some cases a 'trial' may be generated by randomly selecting an individual from the population, as discussed in Chapter 2. For example, the prevalence of diabetes in the population may be 1%, where the prevalence of a disease is the number of people in a population with the disease at a certain time divided by the number of people in the population (see Chapter 9 for further details). If a trial were selected by randomly selecting one person from the population and testing for diabetes, the individual would be expected to be diabetic with probability 0.01. If the sampling of individuals from the population were repeated, the proportion of diabetics in the total sample taken would be expected to be approximately 1%.

However, in some situations the idea of repeated sampling is not appropriate. When the chance of a nuclear reactor melting is specified as less than one in a million per year, the estimate is not based on repeated melt-downs, but rather on the strength of belief of the event happening. When a patient presents with chest pains, a clinician may say that the probability that the patient has heart disease is 20%. However, the individual patient either has or has not got heart disease. The probability is a measure of the strength of the belief of the clinician in the two alternative hypotheses, that the patient has or has not got heart disease. This is termed a *subjective* probability. A clinician will often proceed to further examinations of the patient to modify the strength of his subjective belief that the patient has or has not got heart disease. Thus there are essentially two approaches to probability: a frequency approach and a subjective approach. Most statisticians tend to adopt a frequency approach whereas the nature of diagnostic procedures tends to lead clinicians to a subjective approach. The differences between these two approaches, which are often not explicitly stated, can lead to confusion.

Further concepts concerning probability are introduced in the context of diagnostic tests.

3.2 DIAGNOSTIC TESTS

(a) Uses of a diagnostic test

In making a diagnosis, a clinician establishes a set of diagnostic alternatives and then attempts to reduce these by progressively ruling out specific diseases. Alternatively, the clinician may have a strong hunch that the patient has one particular disease and then sets about confirming it. Given a particular diagnosis, a good test should indicate either that the disease is unlikely or that it is probable. In a practical sense it is important to realise that a diagnostic test is useful only if it influences patient management. If the management is the same for two different diseases, then there is little point in trying strenuously to discriminate between them.

(b) Sensitivity and specificity

Many diagnostic test results are given in the form of a continous variable, such as diastolic blood pressure or haemoglobin count. However, for ease of discussion we will first assume that these have been divided into positive or negative results. Thus a positive result of 'hypertension' is a diastolic blood pressure greater than 90 mmHg; for 'anaemia', a haemoglobin level less than 12 g/dl.

For every laboratory test or diagnostic procedure there is a set of fundamental questions that should be asked. Firstly, if the disease is present, what is the probability that the test result will be positive? This leads to the notion of the *sensitivity* of the test. Secondly, if the disease is absent, what is the probability that the test result will be negative? This question refers to the *specificity* of the test. These questions can only be answered if it is known what the 'true' diagnosis is. In the case of organic disease this can be determined by biopsy or an expensive and risky procedure such as angiography for heart disease. In other cases it may be an 'expert's' opinion. Such tests provide the so-called 'gold standard'.

Example from the literature

Consider the results of an exercise tolerance test on patients with suspected coronary disease obtained by Weiner *et al.* (1979) and summarised in Table 3.1. The disease was diagnosed by angiography and a positive exercise test was defined as more than 1 mm of depression or elevation of part of the ECG during exercise in comparison with the resting baseline recording.

Table 3.1   Results of exercise tolerance test in patients with suspected coronary artery disease

| | | Coronary artery disease | | |
		Present (D+)	Absent (D−)	Total
Exercise	Positive (T+)	815 (e)	115 (g)	930
tolerance	Negative (T−)	208 (f)	327 (h)	535
test				
	Total	1023	442	1465

Source: Weiner *et al.* (1979).

We denote a positive test result by T+, and a positive diagnosis of coronary artery disease by D+. The prevalence of coronary artery disease in these patients is $1023/1465 = 0.70$ or 70%. Thus, the probability of a patient chosen at random from this group having the disease is estimated to be 0.70. We can write this as $P(D+) = 0.70$.

The *sensitivity* of a test is the proportion of those with the disease who also have a positive result. Thus the sensitivity is $e/(e+f) = 815/1023 = 0.80$ or 80%. Now sensitivity is the probability of a positive test result (event T+) given that the disease is present (event D+) and can be written as $P(T+|D+)$, where the | is read as 'given'.

The *specificity* of the test is the proportion of those without the disease who give a negative test result. Thus the specificity is $h/(g + h) = 327/442 = 0.74$ or 74%. Now specificity is the probability of a negative test result (event T−) given that the disease is absent (event D−) and can be written as $P(T-|D-)$.

Since sensitivity is *conditional* on the disease being present and specificity on the disease being absent, in theory, they are unaffected by disease prevalence. For example, if we doubled the number of subjects with true coronary artery disease from 1023 to 2046 in Table 3.1, so that the prevalence was now $2046/(1465+1023) = 82\%$, then we could expect twice as many patients to give a positive test result. Thus $2 \times 815 = 1630$ would have a positive result. In this case the sensitivity would be $1630/2046 = 0.80$, which is unchanged from the previous value. A similar result is obtained for specificity. Sensitivity and specificity are useful statistics because they will yield consistent results for the diagnostic test in a variety of patient groups with different disease prevalences. Although indeed they are independent of disease prevalence, in practice if the disease is very rare, the accuracy with which one can estimate the sensitivity will be strictly limited.

Two other terms in common use are: the *false negative rate* which is given by $f/(e+f) = 1-$ (sensitivity), and the *false positive* rate, or $g/(g + h) = 1-$ (specificity).

3.3 BAYES' THEOREM

(a) Predictive value of a test

Suppose a doctor is confronted by a patient with chest pain suggestive of angina, and that the results of the study described in Table 3.1 are to hand. The doctor therefore believes that the patient has coronary artery disease with probability 0.70. In terms of betting, one would be willing to lay odds of about 7:3 that the patient does have coronary artery disease. The patient now takes the exercise test and the result is positive. How does this modify the odds? It is first necessary to calculate the probability of the patient having the disease, given a positive test result. From Table 3.1, there are 930 men with a positive test, of whom 815 have coronary artery disease. Thus, the estimate of 0.70 for the patient is adjusted upwards to the probability of disease, with a positive test result, of $815/930 = 0.88$.

This gives the *predictive value* of a *positive* test or $P(D+|T+)$. The *predictive value* of a *negative* test is $P(D-|T-)$.

From Table 3.1 the predictive value of a positive exercise tolerance test is $815/930 = 0.88$ and the predictive value of a negative test is $327/535 = 0.61$. These values are affected by the prevalence of the disease. For example, if those with the disease doubled in Table 3.1, then the predictive value of a positive test would then become $1630/(1630 + 115) = 0.93$ and the predictive value of a negative test $416/(327 + 416) = 0.56$.

How does the predictive value $P(D+|T+)$ relate to sensitivity $P(T+|D+)$? Clearly the former is what the clinician requires and the latter is what is supplied with the test. This is discussed in the next section.

(b) Multiplication rule and Bayes' theorem

For any two events A and B, the joint probability of A and B, that is the probability of both A and B occurring simultaneously, is equal to the product of the probability of A given B times the probability of B, thus

$$P(\text{A and B}) = P(\text{A}|\text{B})\, P(\text{B})$$

This is known as the *multiplication* rule of probabilities.

Suppose event A occurs when the exercise test is positive and event B occurs when angiography is positive. The probability of having both a positive exercise test and coronary artery disease is thus $P(\text{T+ and D+})$. From Table 3.1, the probability of picking out one man with both a positive exercise test and coronary heart disease from the group of 1465 men is $815/1465 = 0.56$.

However, from the multiplication rule,

$$P(\text{T+ and D+}) = P(\text{T+}|\text{D+})\, P(\text{D+})$$

$P(\text{T+}|\text{D+}) = 0.80$ is the sensitivity of the test and $P(\text{D+}) = 0.70$ is the prevalence of coronary disease and so $P(\text{T+ and D+}) = 0.80 \times 0.70 = 0.56$, as before.

A moment's thought should convince the reader that it would not matter if the labelling had been reversed, adopting the convention that A occurs when angiography is positive and B occurs when the exercise test is positive, and thus that $P(\text{A and B}) = P(\text{B and A})$. From the multiplication rule it follows that

$$P(\text{AB})\, P(\text{B}) = P(\text{B}|\text{A})\, P(\text{A})$$

This leads to what is known as *Bayes' theorem* or

$$P(\text{B}|\text{A}) = \frac{P(\text{A}|\text{B})\, P(\text{B})}{P(\text{A})}$$

This formula is not appropriate if $P(\text{A}) = 0$, that is if A is an event which cannot happen.

Bayes' theorem enables the predictive value of a positive test to be related to the sensitivity of the test, and the predictive value of a negative test to be related to the specificity of the test. Bayes' theorem enables *prior* assessments about the chances of a diagnosis to be combined with the eventual test results to obtain an *a posteriori* assessment about the diagnosis. It reflects the procedure of making a clinical judgement.

In terms of Bayes' theorem, the diagnostic process is summarised by

$$P(\text{D}+|\text{T}+) = \frac{P(\text{T}+|\text{D}+)\, P(\text{D}+)}{P(\text{T}+)}$$

The probability $P(\text{D}+)$ is the *a priori* probability and $P(\text{D}+|\text{T}+)$ is the *a posteriori* probability. The ratio $P(\text{T+}|\text{D}+)/P(\text{T}+)$ is termed the *likelihood*.

Clearly, most clinicians do not go through the mathematics of the above process, although Macartney (1987) has shown how the formal method closely follows the intuitive approach usually adopted by clinicians. Knill-Jones (1987) gives numerous examples of how the diagnosis of a large number of diseases has been formalised, and adapted for use with a computer.

Example

This example illustrates Bayes' theorem in practice by calculating the positive predictive value for the data of Table 3.1. There, $P(T+) = 930/1465 = 0.63$, $P(D+) = 0.70$ and $P(T+|D+) = 0.80$, thus

$$P(D+|T+) = \frac{\text{Sensitivity} \times \text{Prevalence}}{\text{Probability of positive result}}$$

$$= \frac{P(T+|D+)P(D+)}{P(T+))}$$

$$= \frac{0.80 \times 0.70}{0.63} = 0.88.$$

Example

The prevalence of a disease is 1 in 1000, and there is a test that can detect it with a sensitivity of 100% and specificity of 95%. What is the probability that a person has the disease, given a positive result on the test?

Many people, without thinking, might guess the answer to be 0.95, the specificity. Using Bayes' theorem, however,

$$P(D+|T+) = \frac{\text{Sensitivity} \times \text{Prevalence}}{\text{Probability of a positive result}}$$

To calculate the probability of a positive result consider 1000 people in which 1 person has the diesase. The test will certainly detect this one person. However, it will also give a positive result on 5% of the 999 people without the disease. Thus the total positives is $1 + 0.05 \times 999 = 50.95$ and the probability is $50.95/1000 = 0.05095$.

Thus $$P(D+|T+) = \frac{1 \times 0.001}{0.05095} = 0.02.$$

Two events A and B are *independent* if the fact that B has happened does not influence whether A will occur, that is $P(A|B) = P(A)$. Thus from the multiplication rule two events are independent if $P(A \text{ and } B) = P(A) \times P(B)$.

In Table 3.1, if the results of the exercise tolerance test were totally unrelated to whether or not a patient had coronary artery disease, we might expect

$$P(D+ \text{ and } T+) = P(T+)P(D+)$$

If we estimate $P(D+ \text{ and } T+)$ as $815/1465 = 0.56$, $P(D+) = 1023/1465 = 0.70$ and $P(T+) = 930/1465 = 0.63$ then the difference

$$P(D+ \text{ and } T+) - P(D+)\,P(T+) = 0.56 - 0.70 \times 0.63 = 0.12$$

is a crude measure of whether these events are independent. In this case the size of the difference would suggest they are not independent. The question of deciding whether events are or are not independent belongs to statistical inference and will be discussed in Chapter 6.

The next section generalises Bayes' theorem to the situation where there can be a wider range of outcomes than simply that the patient has or has not got a disease.

(c) Diagnosis with more than two outcomes

To generalise Bayes' theorem we need the concept of mutually exlusive events. Events are *mutually exclusive* if, when one event occurs, the others cannot. Diagnoses are often considered as mutually exclusive. Thus a patient complaining of abdominal pain may have either appendicitis, dyspepsia or colic, but the diagnosis of one precludes the others. Similarly, when a coin is tossed, the event can be either a 'head' or a 'tail' but cannot be both. If two events A and B are mutually exclusive then have the addition rule of mutually exclusive events applies:

$$P(A \text{ or } B) = P(A) + P(B)$$

It also follows that if A and B are mutually exclusive,

$$P(A \text{ and } B) = 0$$

Now consider the situation in which a middle-aged male patient enters the doctor's surgery and complains of pain in the lower part of his chest. Suppose it is known that in every 1000 such patients 5 will have coronary artery disease (CAD), 10 will have chronic obstructive airways disease (COAD) and 50 will have indigestion (I). Suppose further that these diagnoses are mutually exclusive. When questioned, the patient states that the chest pain occurs during exercise and goes away when he stops exercising. The doctor knows that patients with coronary artery disease will certainly experience these symptoms, of those with obstructive airways disease about 20% will complain of these symptoms and that 5% with indigestion will complain of these symptoms. Suppose these are the only three diagnoses possible and label the symptoms 'S'.

What the doctor requires is the probability of CAD, *given* the symptoms S; that is, the conditional probability $P(CADS)$. Using Bayes' theorem,

$$P(CAD|S) = \frac{P(S|CAD)\,P(CAD)}{P(S)}$$

From the above, $P(S|CAD) = 1$ and $P(CAD)$ can be computed because the diagnosis must be one of CAD, COAD or I. Out of 1000 patients only 65 will have one of these diagnoses of which only 5 will have CAD. Thus $P(CAD|CAD \text{ or } COAD \text{ or } I) = 5/65 = 0.08$. How can the value for $P(S)$ be obtained?

Consider a single individual. He either has CAD or COAD or I. Having (S and CAD) is mutually exclusive to having (S and COAD) which is in turn mutually exclusive to having (S and I). The addition rule of mutually exclusive events gives

$P[(S \text{ and } CAD) \text{ or } (S \text{ and } COAD) \text{ or } (S \text{ and } I)]$

$$= P(S \text{ and } CAD) + P(S \text{ and } COAD) + P(S \text{ and } I)$$

The left-hand side of the equation can be written

$$P[S \text{ and } (CAD \text{ or } COAD \text{ or } I)]$$

By the multiplication rule this becomes

$$P(S) \times P[(CAD \text{ or } COAD \text{ or } I)|S]$$

However, the patient must have one of the diagnoses CAD or COAD or I and so

$$P[(CAD \text{ or } COAD \text{ or } I)|S)] = 1$$

Thus

$$P(S) = P(S \text{ and } CAD) + P(S \text{ and } COAD) + P(S \text{ and } I)$$

The multiplication rule can be applied to each one of the terms on the right-hand side of the above equation to get

$$P(S) = P(S|CAD) \, P(CAD) + P(S|COAD) \, P(COAD) + P(S|I) \, P(I)$$

It has already been stated that if the disease is coronary artery disease, then $P(S|CAD) = 1.00$, whereas if the disease is chronic obstructive airway disease, then $P(S|COAD) = 0.20$, and if the disease is indigestion then $P(S|I) = 0.05$. By the multiplication rule, the probability that a patient has the symptoms and coronary artery disease is

$$P(S \text{ and } CAD) \; = \; 1.00 \; \times \; \frac{5}{65} \; = \; 0.08$$

the probability that a patient has the symptoms and chronic obstructive airway disease is

$$P(S \text{ and } COAD) \; = \; 0.20 \; \times \; \frac{10}{65} \; = \; 0.03$$

and the probability that a patient has the symptoms *and* indigestion is

$$P(S \text{ and } I) \; = \; 0.05 \; \times \; \frac{50}{65} \; = \; 0.04$$

Thus

$$P(S) \; = \; 0.08 \; + \; 0.03 \; + \; 0.04 \; = \; 0.15$$

and finally, the probability of coronary artery disease given the symptoms are present is calculated from the formula on the previous page as

$$P(CAD|S) = 1 \times 0.08/0.15 = 0.53$$

Thus the doctor's *a priori* probability of 0.08 that the disease was coronary artery disease has increased to 0.53 but the diagnosis still remains far from certain despite the fact that it was assumed that the question relating to angina is 100% sensitive. Such uncertainty remains because general screening tests are never 100% *specific*, and so the doctor must bear in mind the relative prevalence of different diagnoses before making a final decision. It is a common error when a diagnostic test provides an unexpected result to rely too much on the 'accuracy' of the test when deciding the diagnosis and to ignore the influence of disease prevalence (Parker and Kassiver, 1987).

The process of using diagnostic tests to explore diagnostic hypotheses has strong similarities with the use of statistical tests to explore statistical hypotheses, which will be discussed in Chapter 6.

3.4 RELATIVE (RECEIVER) OPERATING CHARACTERISTICS

When a diagnostic test produces a continuous measurement, then a convenient diagnostic cut-off must be selected to calculate the sensitivity and specificity of the test. Consider the data shown in Table 3.2 on forced expiratory volume (FEV_1) in 40 non-smoking patients with and without coal-workers' pneumoconiosis. The data are expressed as percentages of normal values for a given age and height.

Table 3.2 FEV_1 values (% normal) for subjects with and without coal-workers' pneumoconiosis

Men with pneumoconiosis, $n=27$

40	43	47	49	50	50	53	57	58	58	58	62
65	69	71	73	74	75	75	77	78	79	80	87
90	100	105									

Men without pneumoconiosis, $n=13$

60	67	73	75	79	80	83	87	89
100	105	109	115					

Source: Part data from Musk *et al*. (1981).

For diagnostic purposes a commonly used cut-off value in respiratory medicine is to take 80% of the FEV_1 expected in a healthy person of the same age and height. Applying this cut-off to the data of Table 3.2 gives the 2 × 2 table summary of Table 3.3.

From Table 3.3 the sensitivity is 22/27 = 0.81, or 81%, and the specificity is 8/13 = 0.62, or 62%. By redefining the cut-off point one changes both the sensitivity and specificity.

One way of displaying the ability of a test to discriminate between diseased and healthy groups without having to specify a particular cut-off level is to graph the sensitivity on the *y*-axis against the false positive rate for all possible cut-off values of the diagnostic test on the *x*-axis. The resulting curve is known as the *relative* (or *receiver*) *operating characteristic curve* (ROC) and is shown in Figure 3.1 for the FEV_1 data of Table 3.2.

Table 3.3 FEV_1 above and below 80% normal value by pneumoconiosis status

		Pneumoconiosis		
		Present	Absent	Total
FEV_1	<80% of normal	22	5	27
	≥80% of normal	5	8	13
	Total	27	13	40

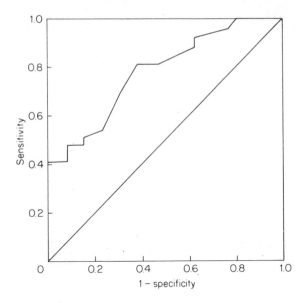

Figure 3.1   An ROC curve for the data in Table 3.2

A perfect diagnostic test would be one with no false positive or false negative results and would be represented by a line that started at the origin and went up the y-axis to a sensitivity of 1, and then horizontally across to a false positive rate of 1. A test that produces a false positive result at the same rate as true positive results would produce an ROC on the diagonal line $y = x$. Any reasonable diagnostic test will display an ROC curve in the upper left triangle of Figure 3.1. When more than one laboratory test is available for the same clinical problem one can compare ROC curves.

Example from the literature

Hannequin *et al*. (1988) describe a study in which they were attempting to discriminate between malignant and benign thyroid nodules (see Figure 3.2). The two tests are either a function of the age and sex of the patient and morphology of the tumour, or these variables plus the result of cytology, where this was available. For a given specificity the result with cytology consistently gives a greater sensitivity, and so including cytology is clearly useful for discriminating between the two groups.

Methods for the statistical comparison of two ROC curves, that is, to help decide whether apparent differences in curves could have arisen by chance, are available but they are complex. A useful discussion is given by Beck and Shultz (1986).

The selection of an optimal combination of sensitivity and specificity for a particular test requires an analysis of the relative medical consequences and costs of false positive and false negative interpretations. Thus the reason for not giving angiographs to all patients with suspected heart disease is that it is a difficult and expensive procedure, and carries a non-negligible risk to the patient. An alternative test such as the exercise test might be tried, and only if it is positive would angiography then be carried out. If the

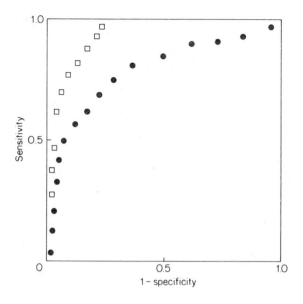

Figure 3.2   ROC curves of tests with (□) and without (●) cytology to discriminate between benign and malignant thyroid tumours (after Hannequin *et al.*, 1988)

exercise test is negative then the next stage would be to carry out biochemical tests, and if these turned out positive, once again angiography could be performed.

3.5 POINTS WHEN READING THE LITERATURE

(1) To whom has the diagnostic test been applied? It is possible that characteristics of the patients or stage and severity of the disease can influence the sensitivity of the test. For example, it is likely that a test for cancer will have greater sensitivity for advanced rather than early disease. Have the authors given enough information to make the disease status clear?

(2) How has the group of patients used in the analysis been selected, and in particular how has the decision to verify the test by the 'gold standard' been made? A common error is to select patients in some manner for verification of a previous diagnosis; this usually leads to positive tests being over-represented in the verified sample and the sensitivity being inflated. It is also common to assume that unverified cases are disease-free, which can lead to inflated specificity estimates. The best way to avoid verification bias is to construct a prospective study in which all patients receive definite verification of disease status.

(3) How have the investigators coped with uninterpretable results; that is, results that one can neither say are positive nor negative? If the reason for uninterpretability is essentially random, and is unrelated to disease status, then the test characteristics can be estimated. If it is related to disease status then the uninterpretable results cannot be safely ignored. In any case, the proportion of uninterpretable results should be

given in any diagnostic test efficacy study, since it is an important consideration in the cost-effectiveness of the test.

(4) Did the investigator who provided the diagnostic test result know other clinical results about the patients? Diagnostic tests are usually carried out during, or in conjunction with, the clinical examination. Where there is an element of subjectivity in a test, such as an ECG stress test, a remarkable improvement in sensitivity can be shown when the investigator is aware of other symptoms of the patient!

(5) Was the reproducibility of the test result determined?

(6) Did the patients who had the test actually benefit as a consequence of the test?

(7) How good is the gold standard? The ideal gold standard either may not exist or be very expensive or invasive and therefore not carried out. In this case, the test used as the gold standard may be subject to error, which, in turn, will bias the estimates of sensitivity and specificity.

Chapter 4

Data description

Summary

This chapter describes methods of graphical and tabular display of data. The different types of data and measures of location and variation are introduced.

4.1 INTRODUCTION

In a survey, experiment or clinical trial, all the information is contained in the measurements made. Suppose it is required to encapsulate this information in order to communicate the results to a colleague or newspaper reporter by telephone. It is hardly feasible to read off a string of data values! Most people cannot cope with large quantities of data. They either require a visual image or a small set of numbers, often termed *statistics*, that will describe the key features of the data. The usual features that are of interest are some measure of location, describing the level of the data values, and some measure of variability, describing how the data values change from subject to subject.

The ability to communicate results efficiently is a vital skill for anyone undertaking studies of any form. This will often be done by means of graphical type figures or tables containing numerical information.

4.2 DATA PRESENTATION

The principal object of data presentation, whether tabular or graphical, is to convey the essential features of a study to any reader of the final publication. It is important that the presentation contains only important information, as editorial restrictions often prevent numerous tables and graphs in any one paper in a scientific journal. However, there are usually many tabulations and graphs to be examined at the analysis stage before a decision can be made on which to present in a final report. Graphical display can also be used to check the assumptions underlying a statistical analysis. For example, graphs can be used to look for unusual observations which may result from recording errors, or observations which are unusually influential on the parameter estimated. Data can be plotted to check if the relationship between two variables is approximately linear or if the distribution of the variable has a Normal distribution form. Approaches to data presentation may depend on the quantity of data available. With very large data sets, individual points on a graph are tedious to plot and difficult to view, whereas with small data sets individual values can be given.

4.3 TYPES OF DATA

Before discussing how data can be displayed, it is first necessary to distinguish between different types of data.

Example from the literature

For illustrative purposes consider the data in Table 4.1, which gives details of 1000 women recruited to a randomised trial by Sleep and Grant (1987), who compared alternative policies with respect to episiotomy during spontaneous vaginal delivery.

Table 4.1 Details of two trial groups comparing two policies with respect to episiotomy

		Questionnaire responders		Questionnaire non-responders	
		Restrictive	Liberal	Restrictive	Liberal
Number of subjects		329	345	169	157
Age	Mean	27.0	27.0	25.9	26.0
(years)	SD	4.9	5.0	5.6	4.2
Primiparous	Number	135	152	66	67
	%	41	44	39	43
Married	Number	300	318	145	117
	%	91	92	86	75
Baby age	Mean	39.8	40.0	39.7	39.5
(weeks)	SD	1.2	1.2	1.3	1.1
Birthweight	Mean	3426	3407	3330	3280
(g)	SD	430	451	475	394
Number (%)	None	102(31)	73(21)	67(40)	49(31)
with	Tear alone	190(58)	92(27)	88(52)	31(20)
posterior	Episiotomy	32(10)	160(46)	13(8)	67(43)
trauma	Episiotomy and extension	5(2)	20(6)	1(1)	10(6)
Number (%) with anterior tears		90(27)	55(16)	41(24)	32(20)

Source: Sleep and Grant (1987).

(a) Qualitative data

(i) Nominal data

Nominal data consist of unordered 'either–or' observations, for example: Dead or Alive; Male or Female; Cured or Not cured; Blood group A, O, B or AB; Pregnant or Not pregnant; Infected or Not infected. The methods of presentation of nominal data are limited in scope. Thus Table 4.1 merely gives the number (or frequency) and percentage (or relative frequency) of married women in each of four groups.

(ii) Ordered classifications

If there are more than two categories of classification it may be possible to order them in some way. For example, after treatment a patient is either improved, the same or worse; a woman may never have conceived, conceived but spontaneously aborted, or given birth to a live infant. Table 4.1 orders the categories of women with posterior trauma in order of severity, from none, through tear alone, episiotomy alone, to episiotomy and extension.

(iii) Ranked data

In some studies it may be appropriate to use classifications that can be ranked. For example, patients with rheumatoid arthritis may be asked to order their preference for four dressing aids. Here although numerical values are assigned to each aid one cannot assume they behave as numbers. They are in fact only codes for best, second best, third best and worst.

(b) Numerical or quantitative data

(i) Numerical discrete

Such data consist of counts; thus the study by Sleep and Grant (1987) also details the number of babies born to the 1000 women over a three-year period.

(ii) Numerical continuous

Such data are measurements that can, in theory at least, take any value within a given range. Examples in Table 4.1 are maternal age, gestational age and birthweight of baby.

4.4 SUMMARISING DATA

(a) Measures of location

(i) Mean or average

The *mean* or average of *n* observations is simply the sum of the observations divided by their number, thus

$$\bar{x} = \frac{\text{Sum of all sample values}}{\text{Size of sample}} = \frac{\Sigma x}{n}$$

Here x represents the individual sample values and Σx their sum. In Table 4.1, the mean weight of the 329 babies born to the restrictive policy group who are questionnaire responders is 3426 g. The major advantage of the mean is that it uses all the data values, and is, in a statistical sense, efficient. The mean also characterises some important statistical distributions to be discussed in Chapter 5. Its main disadvantage is that it is vulnerable to what are known as *outliers*. Outliers are single observations which if excluded from the calculations have noticeable influences on the results. It does not necessarily follow that they should be excluded from the final data summary, or that they result from an erroneous measurement.

(ii) Median and quartiles

The *quartiles*, *lower*, *median* and *upper*, are values of the variable which divide the distribution into four parts of equal area. They are estimated from the data by first ordering the data from smallest to largest and then counting upwards the appropriate number of observations. The estimate of, for example, the median or middle quartile, is either the observation at the centre of the ordering in the case of an odd number of observations, or the simple average of the 'middle' two observations if the total number of observations is even. The quartiles are calculated in a similar way. The median has the advantage that it is not affected by outliers. However, it is not statistically efficient as it does not make use of all the individual data values.

(b) Measures of dispersion or variability

(i) Range and inter-quartile range

The *range* is calculated as the largest minus the smallest observation. The *inter-quartile range* is the difference between the upper and lower quartiles. The range is vulnerable to outliers whereas the inter-quartile range is not.

(ii) Standard deviation

The *standard deviation* is calculated as follows:

$$s = \sqrt{\frac{\Sigma(x - \bar{x})^2}{n - 1}}$$

The expression $\Sigma(x - \bar{x})^2$ is interpreted as follows: from each x-value subtract the mean $\bar{x}$, square this difference, then add each of the n squared differences. This sum is then divided by $(n - 1)$ and finally the square root is taken to give the standard deviation. Thus the standard deviation of the weight of 329 babies referred to above is 430 g. It turns out in many situations that about 95% of observations will be within 2 standard deviations of the mean. For this example, this implies that the majority of babies will be between 2566 and 4286 g (more sensibly rounded to between 2550 and 4300 g). Standard deviation is often abbreviated to SD in the medical literature. It will be denoted here as SD(x), where the bracketed x is emphasised for a reason to be introduced later. The *variance* is the square of the standard deviation.

4.5 VARIABILITY

(a) Within-subject variability

Example from the literature

Figure 4.1 shows an example in which low back pain, assessed using a visual analogue scale (VAS) by the patient, is measured on a daily basis for a pre-treatment week, and thereafter during the course of a placebo treatment for four weeks. Details of the study are given in Machin, Lewith and Wylson (1988).

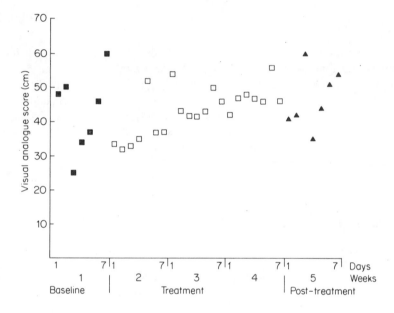

Figure 4.1   Visual analogue pain scores recorded on a daily basis by one patient with low back pain receiving placebo therapy (after Machin *et al.*, 1988)

The observed scores are subject to random fluctuations. The patient illustrated was receiving no active therapy; nevertheless there is considerable day-to-day variation but little evidence of any trend over time. Such variation is termed *within-subject* variation. Within-subject variation is unlikely to be independent, that is, successive values will be dependent on values preceding them. For example, when a patient is in remission then if pain, as recorded by the VAS, is low on one day it is likely to be low the next. This does not imply that the pain will be low, only that it is a good bet that it will be. In contrast examples can be found in which low values are usually followed by high values and vice versa. With independent observations the value on one day gives no indication or clue as to the value on the next.

It is clear from Figure 4.1 that the pain levels are not constant over the observation period. This is nearly always the case when medical observations or measurements are taken over time. Such variation occurs for a variety of reasons. For example, pain levels may depend critically on when the patient last received an analgesic or even on the time of day if some diurnal rhythm is influencing levels. In addition, there may be variability in the actual measurement of pain levels, induced possibly by the patient's perception of pain itself being subject to variation. There may be observer-to-observer variation if the successive pain levels were recorded by different nursing personnel rather than the patient. The possibility of recording errors in the laboratory, transcription errors when conveying the results to the clinic or for statistical analysis, should not be overlooked in appropriate circumstances. When only a single observation is made on one patient at one time only, then the influences of the above sources of variation are not assessable, but may nevertheless all be reflected to some extent in the final entry in the patient record.

Suppose successive observations on a patient taken over time fluctuate around some more or less constant level, then the particular level may be influenced by factors within the patient. For example, levels may be affected by the presence of a viral infection whose presence is unrelated to the cause of the low back pain itself. Levels may also be influenced by the severity of the underlying condition and whether concomitant treatment is necessary for the patient. Levels could also be influenced by environmental factors under control of the patient, for example, alcohol and tobacco consumption and diet, and by factors beyond the control of the patient such as age, sex and ethnic origin. The cause of some of the variation in pain levels may be identified and its effect on the variability estimated. Other variation may have no obvious explanation and is usually termed *random* variation. This does not necessarily imply there is no cause of this component of the variation, but rather that its cause has not been identified or is being ignored.

(b) Between-subject variability

Successive patients with low back pain observed in the same way may have differing average levels of pain from each other but with similar patterns of variation about these levels. The variation in mean pain levels from patient to patient is termed *between-subject variability*.

Observations between subjects are usually regarded as independent. That is, the data values on one subject are not influenced by those obtained from another. This, however, may not always be the case, particularly with subjective measures in which different patients may collaborate in recording their pain levels.

In the investigation of total variability it is very important to distinguish within-subject from between-subject variability. Between- and within-subject variation will always be present in any biological material, whether animals, healthy subjects, patients or histological sections. The experimenter must be aware of possible sources which contribute to the variation, decide on which are of importance in the intended study, and design the study appropriately.

4.6 DISPLAYING DATA

(a) Dot plots

Example from the literature

Figure 4.2 shows a dot plot modified from that of Milsom *et al.* (1987) to illustrate the distribution of strontium concentration in extracellular fluid in three groups of subjects.

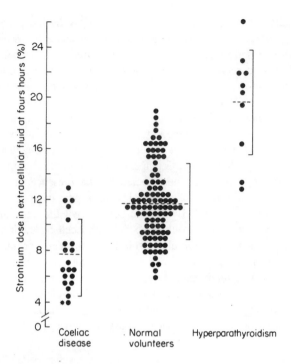

Figure 4.2 Four-hour strontium concentrations in normal volunteers, patients with coeliac disease and patients with primary hyperparathyroidism (after Milsom *et al.*, 1987, with permission)

Here strontium concentration is a continuous variable, and group membership of coeliac, normal or hyperparathyroidism, is a nominal variable. This method of presentation retains the individual subject values and clearly demonstrates differences between the groups in a readily appreciated manner. An additional advantage is that any outliers will be detected by such a plot. However, such presentation is not usually practical with large numbers of subjects in each group.

Dot plots can be of particular value if observations on experimental units are repeated on more than one occasion, for example, before and after treatment with a particular drug. In such a situation the associated, or paired, dots are joined.

Example from the literature

Cohen, Dodds and Viberti (1987) link the glomerular filtration rates in seven insulin-dependent diabetics when fed on normal and low-protein diets in Figure 4.3.

The figure indicates a small but consistently lower level in all subjects when they received the low-protein diet, which would not have been apparent if the dots had not been so joined.

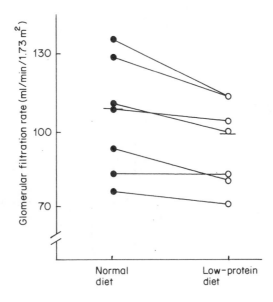

Figure 4.3 Glomerular filtration rate during normal and low-protein diets in insulin dependent diabetics (after Cohen *et al.*, 1987, with permission)

(b) Histograms

Patterns in large data sets may be revealed by forming a histogram. This is obtained by first dividing up the range of a numerically continuous variable into several non-overlapping and equal intervals or classes, then counting the number of observations in each interval. Thus for the normal volunteers of Figure 4.2 the dose scale could be divided into groups of 2% intervals giving the histogram of counts as in Figure 4.4.

The area of each histogram block is proportional to the number of subjects in the particular strontium concentration group. Thus the total area in the histogram represents the total number of volunteers. Relative frequency histograms allow comparison between histograms made up of different numbers of observations which may be useful when studies are compared. Numerical discrete data can also be summarised in histogram form by grouping into appropriate intervals. However, if the individual values are presented then it is better to put vertical spikes at each value (rather than blocks) proportional in length to the number of observations (or relative frequency) of each value.

One important reason for producing dot plots and histograms is to get some idea of the shape of the distribution of the data, a point we will come to later. The choice of the number of intervals is important. Too few intervals and much important information may be smoothed out; too many intervals and the underlying shape will be obscured by a mass of confusing detail. It is usual to choose between 5 and 15 intervals, but the correct choice will be based partly a subjective impression of the resulting histogram. Histograms with unequal intervals can be constructed but they are usually best avoided.

Sometimes it is useful to display data in such a way that one can easily tell whether the distribution is close to what is known as 'Normal' (see Section 5.2). One efficient

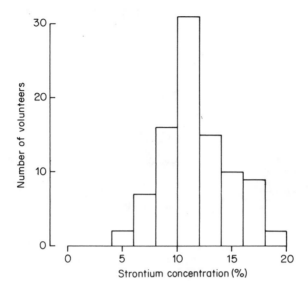

Figure 4.4   Histogram of four-hour strontium concentration in 97 normal volunteers (source: Milsom *et al.*, 1987, with permission)

method of doing this is by means of a Normal probability plot, which is described in detail in Appendix A16.

Example from the literature

Tippett *et al.* (1982) display a Normal probability plot of log serum creatinine kinase (CK) activity in carriers of Duchenne muscular dystrophy and controls. The results are displayed in Figure 4.5.

One can see from the figure that the distribution of log CK activity is close to Normal for the controls because the points are close to a straight line. For carriers the distribution is not quite so close. The variability is considerably greater for carriers because the slope of the line, which is inversely proportional to the standard deviation, is not as steep for carriers as for controls.

(c) Box–whisker plot

If the number of points is large, a dot plot can be replaced by a *box–whisker* plot. Such a plot is more compact than the corresponding histogram. One such plot is illustrated in Figure 4.6, which is again for the normal volunteers of Figure 4.2.

The minimum and maximum values of the variable under consideration are indicated by the extremities (the 'whiskers') of the diagram. The median value is indicated by the central vertical line and the lower and upper quartiles by the corresponding vertical ends of the box. The box–whisker plot as used here therefore displays the median and two

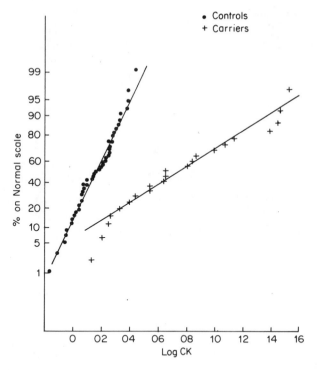

Figure 4.5 Normal probability plot of log CK activity for controls and carriers of Duchenne muscular dystrophy (after Tippett *et al.*, 1982, with permission)

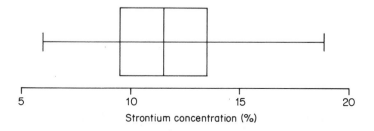

Figure 4.6 Box–whisker plot of strontium concentrations in 97 normal volunteers (source: Milsom *et al.*, 1987, with permission)

measures of spread, namely the range and inter-quartile range. Alternatively it could be constructed to indicate the mean and two SDs either side of the mean.

(d) Time series

In many studies individual patients are monitored over time, as in the example of the patient in Figure 4.1. A common method of presenting observed values during treatment is to express these as a percentage of pre-treatment or baseline scores. For this example, the mean baseline score, that is the mean of the observations for the seven days before the placebo is taken, is 42.9 mm. There is considerable variation about this value, however. This illustrates that calculating successive ratios of daily treatment values of either the day 7 baseline of 60.0 mm or the mean baseline score of 42.9 mm, would give totally different impressions of the patient profile. If the baseline value used happens to be low (or high) for no other reason than random variation, then all successive ratios will be consequently inflated (or diminished). The hazards of the analysis of this type of study are further discussed in Chapter 10.

(e) Scatter plots

The association between quantitative variables can be investigated by means of a *scatter plot*.

Example from the literature

Figure 4.7 shows a scatter plot produced by Soothill, Nicholaides and Campbell (1987) of severity of hypercapnia against severity of hypoxia in 38 foetuses.

It is clear that the severity of hypercapnia and hypoxia are associated in that high values of one are associated with high values of the other. In other contexts scatter plots may show no evidence of association. In Figure 4.7 it is immaterial which variable (hypercapnia or hypoxia) is plotted on which axis. However, if one variable, x, clearly causes the other, y, then it is usual to plot the x variable on the horizontal axis and the y variable on the vertical axis. Thus if a drug is given in various doses, the doses would be along the x-axis and the response measure on the y-axis.

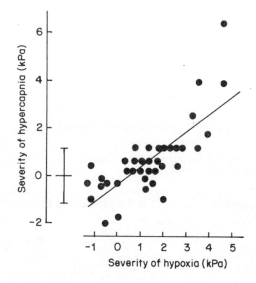

Figure 4.7   Scatter diagram of severity of hypercapnia and hypoxia in 38 growth-retarded foetuses (after Soothill *et al.*, 1987, with permission)

Example from the literature

Such an example is given by Hindmarsh and Brook (1987) who investigate the change in height velocity standard deviation score to growth hormone dose (unit/m³/week) given to children of short stature but otherwise normal (Figure 4.8).

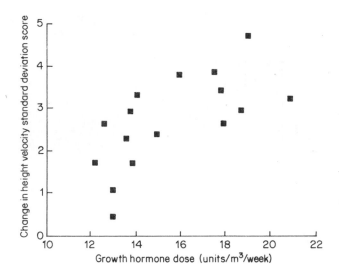

Figure 4.8   Relation between dose of growth hormone and change in height velocity standard deviation score over one year (after Hindmarsh and Brook, 1987, with permission)

(f) Survival curves

In a study of patients with early breast cancer, the time from surgery to recurrence of the disease may be of interest. For those women who have had a recurrence, the recurrence-free survival is measured as the number of days from surgery to the recurrence. For those women who have had the surgery but not yet the recurrence, the number of days from operation to the time the patient was last examined can be calculated. However, since the recurrence has not yet occurred, all we can say is that her recurrence-free survival is at least as long as the interval so calculated. The recurrence-free survival so observed is termed *censored*. For example, if the time post surgery is 130 weeks without recurrence the recurrence-free survival is then conventionally denoted as 130+ weeks. In addition, some may die without recurrence of their disease and for reasons unrelated to the disease. Such women would also generate censored recurrence-free survival times. Many subjects in this type of study are likely to have censored observations unless the investigator waits until they all fail (that is, in this case, until the disease recurs) and does not recruit more subjects in the meantime. Thus, at analysis, the time to recurrence in 10 women may be 2, 3, 6+, 7, 8+, 10, 10+, 12 and 15 years.

Example from the literature

An example of censored survival times, which are indicated by arrows in Figure 4.9, is given by McIllmurray and Turkie (1987).

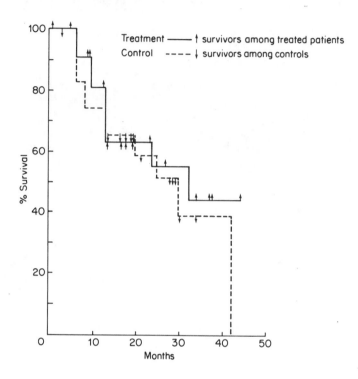

Figure 4.9 Survival curves for patients with Dukes's C rectal cancer by placebo and γ-linolenic acid groups (after McIllmurray and Turkie, 1987, with permission)

They show the life table survival rates of patients receiving control or γ-linolenic acid treatment in patients with Dukes's C colorectal cancer.

Life table calculations are described in Appendix A17.

4.7 PRESENTATION

(a) Graphs

In any graph there are clearly certain items that are important. For example, scales should be labelled clearly with appropriate dimensions added. The plotting symbols are also important; a graph is used to give an impression of pattern in the data, so bold and relatively large plotting symbols are desirable. By all means identify the position of the point with a fine pen but mark it so others can see. This is particularly important if it is to be reduced for publication purposes or presented as a slide in a talk. A graph should never include too much clutter, for example, many overlapping groups each with a different symbol. In such a case it is usually preferable to give a series of graphs, albeit smaller, in several panels. The choice of scales for the axes will depend on the particular data set. If transformations of the axes are used, for example, plotting on a log scale, it is usually better to mark the axes using the original scale as this will be more readily understood by the reader. Breaks in scales should be avoided. If breaks are unavoidable under no circumstances must points on either side of a break be joined. If both axes have the same units, then use the same scale for each. If this cannot be done easily, it is sensible to indicate the line of equality, perhaps feintly, in the figure. False impression of trend, or lack of it, in a time plot can sometimes be introduced by omitting the zero point of the vertical axis. There must always be a compromise between clarity of reproduction, that is filling the space available with data points, and clarity of message. Appropriate measures of variability should also be included. One such is to indicate the range of values covered by two standard deviations either side a plotted mean.

With currently available microcomputer graphics packages one can now perform extensive exploration of the data, not only to determine more carefully their structure, but also to find the best means of summary and presentation. This is usually worth considerable effort.

(b) Tables

Although graphical presentation is very desirable it should not be overlooked that tabular methods are very important (see Table 4.1). In particular, tables can give more precise numerical information than a graph, for example the number of observations, the mean and some measure of variability of each tabular entry. They often take less space than a graph containing the same information. Standard statistical computer packages can be easily programmed to provide basic summary statistics in tabular form on many variables.

4.8 POINTS WHEN READING THE LITERATURE

(1) Is the number of subjects involved clearly stated?
(2) Has account been taken of any pairing of data?
(3) Are appropriate axes clearly labelled and scales indicated?
(4) Do the titles adequately describe the contents of the tables and graphs?
(5) Are appropriate measures of location and variation used in the paper?
(6) Do the graphs indicate the relevant variability?

Chapter 5

From sample to population

Summary

In this chapter the concepts of a population and its associated parameters are described. The sample from a population is used to provide the estimates of the population parameters. The importance of the Normal distribution is stressed. The standard error is introduced and methods for calculating confidence intervals for population means for continuous data having a Normal distribution and for discrete data which follow binomial or Poisson distributions are given.

5.1 INTRODUCTION

In the statistical sense a *population* is a theoretical concept used to describe an entire group. Examples are the population of all patients with diabetes mellitus, or the population of all middle-aged men. *Parameters* are quantities used to describe characteristics of such populations. Thus the proportion of diabetic patients with nephropathy, or the mean blood pressure of middle-aged men are characteristics describing the two populations. *Samples* are taken from populations to provide *estimates* of population parameters.

In many medical investigations, whether a laboratory experiment, clinical trial or epidemiological study, the purpose of summarising the behaviour of a particular group is usually to draw some inference about a wider population of which the group is a sample. For example, a group of volunteers are investigated to help determine a *reference* or *normal range* for a certain laboratory test. The object is to use the resultant reference interval as that for the healthy population as a whole. The presence of a suspected disease in a patient is then indicated if the corresponding test value lies outside this reference interval. It is clearly important that the 'volunteers' are chosen carefully so that they do reflect the population as a whole and not a particular subset of that population. If the volunteers are selected at random from the population then the calculated reference interval will be an estimate of the reference interval or normal range of the population. Clearly, the larger the sample, the better the estimate. It is important to note that populations are unique, but that samples are not. Thus for middle-aged men there is only one normal range for blood pressure. However, one investigator taking a random sample from a population of healthy middle-aged men and measuring their blood pressure will obtain a different normal range to another investigator who takes a different random sample from the same population of such men.

5.2 THE NORMAL DISTRIBUTION

It is often the case with medical data that the histogram of a continuous variable obtained from a single measurement on different subjects will have a characteristic 'bell-shaped' distribution. One such example is the histogram of the logarithm of the urine sugar levels in 840 patients with diabetes mellitus shown in Figure 5.1.

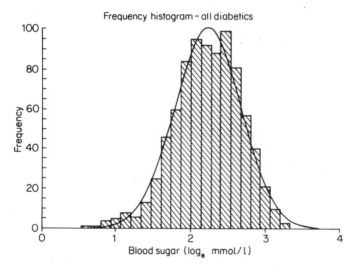

Figure 5.1 Distribution of urine sugar levels in non-diabetic subjects (data obtained by Gatling, Mullee and Hill, 1988)

In fact the histogram of the actual urine sugar levels in these patients was not symmetric. The right-hand tail of the distribution was much longer than the left-hand tail. Such a distribution is termed *skew* to the right. A distribution with a relatively longer left-hand tail is termed skew to the left. Taking the logarithm of the urine sugar values *transformed* the measure and the histogram on this *transformed scale* appears to have the Normal distribution shape. It is surprising how often a skew distribution can be transformed in this way, either by taking logarithms as in this case, or working with the square root of the variable under consideration. Of course, this will not be always the case and the steps necessary to deal with such circumstances are introduced later.

To distinguish the use of the same word in *normal* range and *Normal* distribution we have used a lower and upper-case convention throughout this book.

The histogram of the sample data is an estimate of the population distribution of urine sugar levels of diabetic patients. This population distribution can be estimated by the superimposed smooth 'bell-shaped' curve or 'Normal' distribution shown. We presume that if we were able to look at the entire population of diabetic patients then the distribution would have exactly the Normal shape. We often infer, from a sample whose histogram has the approximate Normal shape, that the population will have exactly, or as near as makes no practical difference, that Normal shape.

The Normal distribution is completely described by two parameters μ and σ, where μ represents the population mean or centre of the distribution and σ the population standard deviation. As μ changes, the distribution moves along the measurement axis. Populations with small values of the standard deviation σ have a distribution concentrated close to the centre, μ; those with large standard deviation have a distribution widely spread along the measurement axis. One mathematical property of the Normal distribution is that exactly 95% of the distribution lies between

$$\mu - 1.96 \times \sigma \quad \text{and} \quad \mu + 1.96 \times \sigma$$

Changing the multiplier 1.96 to 2.58, exactly 99% of the Normal distribution lies in the corresponding interval. Table T1 shows how the area between various multipliers changes, although this table actually specifies the proportion of the total area, denoted α, in the two tails of the distribution. The proportion of the area between the multipliers is then calculated as $1 - \alpha$.

In practice the two parameters of the Normal distribution, μ and σ, must be estimated from the sample data. For this purpose a random sample from the population is first taken. The sample mean $\bar{x}$ and the sample standard deviation, $SD(x) = s$, are then calculated as described in Chapter 4. If a sample is taken from such a Normal distribution, and, provided the sample is not too small, then approximately 95% of the sample will be covered by

$$\bar{x} - 1.96 \times SD(x) \quad \text{to} \quad \bar{x} + 1.96 \times SD(x)$$

This is calculated by merely replacing the population parameters μ and σ by the sample estimates $\bar{x}$ and s in the previous expression.

In appropriate circumstances this interval may estimate the reference interval for a particular laboratory test which is then used for diagnostic purposes.

Example from the literature

Jung et al. (1988) give the mean and standard deviation for the excretions of the tubular enzyme alanine amniopeptidase (AAP) in 30 healthy male hospital staff members as 1.05 U and 0.32 U respectively. They note that 19 patients with diabetes, without nephropathy, had a higher mean of 1.48 U (SD = 0.49 U) and 17 diabetic patients with nephropathy an even higher mean of 4.45 U (SD = 6.51 U).

Assuming a Normal distribution for AAP in the hospital staff, a reference interval for healthy males would be estimated as 0.44 to 1.69 U. This may then be taken as indicating the range of AAP in which the majority, approximately 95%, of healthy subjects in the wider population will lie. Since patients with diabetes appear to have higher mean AAP levels than healthy individuals, a patient may be investigated for the presence of diabetes by means of AAP levels. A high value, in particular one above the upper reference range limit of 1.69 U, may be taken as an indication of the presence of diabetes. In fact it is possible to calculate what proportion of patients with diabetes will have AAP levels above 1.69 U. To do this, we ask, 'How many standard deviations is 1.69 U above 1.48 U, the mean for the diabetic patients?' Thus we calculate k, where $1.69 = 1.48 + k \times 0.49$ and 0.49 is the sample SD of the diabetics investigated by Jung *et al.* From this we obtain $k = 0.43$. Making use of Table T1 we see that a value of $z = 0.43$ along the axis of the Normal distribution leaves approximately 0.6672 of the distribution in the tails. Hence the proportion in each tail will be $0.6672/2 = 0.3336$. The proportion above the value of 1.69 U is therefore approximately one-third. Thus if we used the upper reference limit of 1.69 U to define the boundary of healthy or 'normality', in the clinical sense, approximately two-thirds of the patients with diabetes will be classed as 'normal'. The *false negative rate*, that is the proportion or percentage of patients assumed to be healthy who are not, is therefore very high at 67%.

The high SD in those subjects with nephropathy as compared to their mean value, indicates the distribution of levels within this group is not symmetric about its centre. This is because if 1.96 standard deviations are subtracted from the corresponding mean we obtain

$$4.45 - (1.96 \times 6.51) = -8.31$$

A negative value for AAP is not possible! Such a situation arises if there are a few individuals in the sample with very high AAP levels compared with the remainder. In this particular case a Normal distribution cannot be assumed to adequately describe the corresponding histogram.

5.3 THE STANDARD ERROR

The above example shows that there is considerable scope for between-subject variation in AAP levels in healthy volunteers. The reference limits are, by definition, a little under four standard deviations apart. The upper reference limit, in this example, is also four times the lower reference limit, yet two patients with such values are both 'normal' in the sense used here. That is they would both fall (just) within the normal reference interval.

Suppose a second group of healthy males is to be investigated to determine AAP levels, comprising individuals from a different hospital from those used for estimating the reference interval. Then provided the particular hospital does not influence mean AAP levels of its volunteers, although individual values may vary considerably from subject to subject, we would not expect the mean value obtained from this new group to be far from that obtained in the first sample.

Fortunately the precision with which a population mean is estimated is measured by the standard deviation of the mean, $SD(\bar{x})$, more commonly referred to as the *standard error of the mean*, $SE(\bar{x})$, or more briefly by SE. This standard error is calculated by dividing the standard deviation by the square root of the number of subjects making up the sample. Here $SE(\bar{x}) = SD(x)/\sqrt{n} = s/\sqrt{n}$.

For the healthy volunteers measured by Jung *et al.* (1988), $n = 30$, $\bar{x} = 1.05$, $s = 0.32$ and $SD(\bar{x}) = 0.32/\sqrt{30} = 0.058$. The bracketed x or $\bar{x}$ after SD emphasise that it is important to use the term 'standard deviation' with some care. Every estimate of a population parameter has its own standard deviation. There is often confusion between the standard error and standard deviation. The standard error always refers to an estimate of a parameter. As such the estimate gets more precise as the number of observations gets larger, which is reflected by the standard error becoming smaller. If the term standard deviation is used in the same way, then it is synonymous with the standard error. However, if it refers to the observations then it is an estimate of the population standard deviation and does not get smaller as the sample size increases.

5.4 CONFIDENCE INTERVALS

Confidence intervals define a range of values within which our population mean μ is likely to lie. Such an interval is defined by

$$\bar{x} - 1.96 \times SD(\bar{x}) \quad \text{to} \quad \bar{x} + 1.96 \times SD(\bar{x})$$

and, in this case, is termed a 95% confidence interval. This is because in Table T1, if $z = 1.96$ then $\alpha = 0.05$, which is $1 - 0.95$. To link z with the corresponding α we write $z_{0.05} = 1.96$. Using the data of the normal volunteers from Jung et al. (1988) gives for this interval 0.94 to 1.16 U. We infer, therefore, that the population mean, μ, is likely to take a value somewhere between 0.94 and 1.16 U. If we had to place bets on a particular value for μ we would bet on one close to the centre of this interval. We would also anticipate other studies in similar patients to have a sample mean within this interval. We would also expect, with our knowledge of the normal range as 0.44–1.69 U, that many patient AAP values would lie outside this confidence interval. The confidence interval is clearly much narrower than the corresponding reference interval. In strict terms the confidence interval is a range of values that is likely to cover the true but unknown population value. The confidence interval is based on the concept of repetition of the study under consideration. Thus if the study were to be repeated 100 times, of the 100 resulting 95% confidence intervals, we would expect 95 of these to include the population parameter. A reported confidence interval from a particular study may or may not include the actual population value.

5.5 THE BINOMIAL DISTRIBUTION

If a group of patients is given a new drug for the relief of a particular condition, then the proportion p being successively treated can be regarded as estimating the population treatment success rate π. The sample proportion p is analogous to the sample mean $\bar{x}$, in that if a score of zero is given to those S patients who fail on treatment, and unity for those R who succeed, then $p = R/n$, where $n = R + S$ is the total number of patients treated. Thus p also represents a mean. We can therefore use a similar expression for a confidence interval for π as we used for μ. The approximate 95% confidence interval for π is given by

$$p - 1.96 \times SD(p) \quad \text{to} \quad p + 1.96 \times SD(p)$$

It turns out that the standard deviation of p is estimated by

$$SD(p) = \sqrt{(pq/n)}$$

where $q = 1 - p$ is the proportion of patients being unsuccessfully treated. Here SD(p) is usually termed the standard error or SE(p).

Example from the literature

Dowson, Lewith and Machin (1985) give the response rate to acupuncture treatment in 25 patients with headache as 32%.

From their data we have $p = 0.32$, SE(p) $= \sqrt{(0.32 \times 0.68/25)} = 0.09$, giving a 95% confidence interval for π as 0.14 to 0.50, that is from 14 to 50%. Although individual patients must score either 0 or 1 according to their treatment outcome, that is they always score a value which lies outside the confidence interval, it is likely that a second group of 25 such patients will have an average response covered by the confidence interval. It should be noted that the confidence interval obtained from the above study covers a very wide range of possible values for the population value π.

Data which can take only a 0 or 1 response, such as treatment failure or treatment success, follow the *binomial distribution* providing the underlying population response rate does not change. The shape of the binomial distribution depends only on π. Suppose $n = 20$ patients are to be treated, and it is known that on average $\pi = 0.25$ will respond to this particular treatment. The number of responses actually observed can take only integer values between 0 (no responses) and 20 (all respond). The binomial distribution for this case is illustrated in Figure 5.2.

The distribution is not symmetric: it has a maximum at 5 responses and the height of the spikes corresponds to the probability of obtaining the particular number of responses from the 20 patients yet to be treated. It should be noted that the expected value for R, the number of successes yet to be observed if n patients are treated, is $n\pi$. The potential

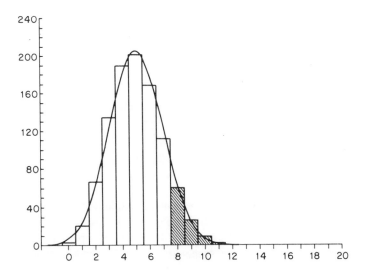

Figure 5.2   Binomial distribution for $n = 20$ with $\pi = 0.25$ and the Normal approximation

variation about this expectation is expressed by the corresponding standard deviation $SD(R) = \sqrt{[n\pi(1 - \pi)]}$.

The reason that a similar expression for the 95% confidence interval for the binomial parameter π can be used as for the Normal distribution parameter μ is illustrated in Figure 5.2. This shows the Normal distribution arranged to have $\mu = n\pi = 5$ and $\sigma = \sqrt{[n\pi(1 - \pi)]} = 1.94$, superimposed onto a binomial distribution with $\pi = 0.25$ and $n = 20$. The Normal distribution describes fairly precisely the binomial distribution in this case.

If n is small, however, or π close to 0 or 1, the disparity between the Normal and binomial distributions with the same mean and standard deviation, similar to those illustrated in Figure 5.2, increases and the Normal distribution can no longer be used to approximate the binomial distribution. In such cases the probabilities generated by the binomial distribution itself must be used. The binomial probabilities are calculated from

$$\text{Prob}(R \text{ responses out of } n) = \frac{n!}{R!(n - R)!} \pi^R (1 - \pi)^{n-R}$$

for successive values of R from 0 through to n. In the above $n!$ is read as n factorial and $R!$ as R factorial. For $R = 4$, $R! = 4 \times 3 \times 2 \times 1 = 24$. Both 0! and 1! are taken as equal to unity. The shaded area marked in Figure 5.2 corresponds to the above expression for the binomial distribution calculated for each of $R = 8, 9, \ldots, 20$ and then added. This area totals 0.1018. This is clearly a tedious calculation to perform although tables are given in, for example, Lindley and Scott (1984). The corresponding area under the approximating Normal distribution is 0.0983. Thus it can be seen that in this case the Normal distribution approximates the binomial probability to 2 decimal places.

It is also only in situations in which reasonable agreement exists between the distributions that we would use the confidence interval expression given previously. For technical reasons, the expression given for a confidence interval for π is an approximation. The approximation will usually be quite good provided π is not too close to 0 or 1, situations in which either almost none or nearly all of the patients respond to treatment. The approximation improves with increasing sample size n. Exact confidence intervals can be calculated using the individual terms of the binomial distribution.

5.6 THE POISSON DISTRIBUTION

Example from the literature

Gore and Altman (1982) quote the data of Thakur, Sharma and Akhtar (1981) summarised in Table 5.1. They recorded the number of patients admitted with acute poisoning to a hospital on each of 49 successive days of full moon.

Now it is clear that the distribution of number of admissions takes integer values only, thus the distribution is similar in this respect to the binomial. However, there is no theoretical limit to the number of admissions that could be made on a particular day although, in practice, no day had more than three such admissions. The situation in which the *Poisson* distribution arises is one in which there is a very large population, here the population of a particular Indian city, each member of which can be thought to have a very small

Table 5.1   Cases of acute poisoning on 49 days of full moon

	Number of hospital admissions					Total number of days
	0	1	2	3	4+	
Observed frequency	16	23	8	2	0	49

Source: Thakur *et al.* (1981).

probability of actually suffering an event, in this case being admitted to hospital with acute poisoning.

The mean admission rate per full-moon day is calculated as

$$r = \frac{(16 \times 0) + (23 \times 1) + (8 \times 2) + (2 \times 3)}{16 + 23 + 8 + 2}$$

$$= \frac{45}{49}$$

$$= 0.92 \text{ admissions per day}$$

It should be noted that the expression for the mean is similar to that for $\bar{x}$ in Chapter 4, except here multiple data values are common, and so instead of writing each as a distinct figure in the numerator they are first grouped and counted. For data arising from a Poisson distribution the standard error, that is the standard deviation of r, is estimated by $SE(r) = \sqrt{(r/n)}$, where n is the total number of admissions. Provided the admission rate is not too low, a 95% confidence interval for the underlying admission rate r can be calculated by

$$r - 1.96 \times SE(r) \quad \text{to} \quad r + 1.96 \times SE(r)$$

In the above example $r = 0.92$, $SE(r) = \sqrt{(r/n)} = \sqrt{(0.92/49)} = 0.12$ and therefore the 95% confidence interval for r is 0.68 to 1.16 admissions per day.

5.7 POINTS WHEN READING THE LITERATURE

(1) What is the population from which the sample was taken? Are there any possible sources of bias that may effect the estimates of the population parameters?
(2) Have reference ranges been calculated on a random sample of healthy volunteers? If not, how does this affect the interpretation? Is there any good reason why a random sample was not taken?
(3) For any continuous variable, are the variables correctly assumed to have a Normal distribution? If not, how do the investigators take account of this?
(4) Has a Normal approximation been used to calculate confidence intervals for a binomial proportion or Poisson rate? If so, is this justified?
(5) It is usual, but not mandatory, to calculate 95% confidence intervals. Have other interval percentages been used?

(6) When authors give the background information to a study they often quote figures of the form $a \pm b$. Although it is usual that a represents the value of the sample mean, if is not always clear what b is. When the intent is to describe the variability found in the sample then b should be the standard deviation. When the intent is to describe the precision of the mean then b should be the standard error.

Chapter 6

Statistical inference

Summary

The concepts of the null hypothesis, statistical significance, the use of statistical tests, p-values and their relation to confidence intervals are introduced. The chapter describes how methods require modification if sample sizes are small or if the data cannot reasonably be assumed to be Normally distributed. The concept of statistical power is discussed. An explanation of the concept of degrees of freedom is given.

6.1 INTRODUCTION

In sampling from a population which can be assumed to have a Normal distribution the sample mean can be regarded as estimating the corresponding population mean μ. Similarly, s estimates the population standard deviation σ. We therefore describe the distribution of the population with the information given by the sample statistics $\bar{x}$ and s. More generally, in comparing two populations, perhaps the population of subjects exposed to a particular hazard and the population of those who were not, two samples are taken, and their respective summary statistics calculated. We might wish to compare the two samples and ask: 'Could they both come from the same population?' That is, does the fact that some subjects have been exposed to the hazard and others not, influence the characteristic or variable we are observing? If it does not, then we regard the two populations as if they were one with respect to the particular variable under consideration.

6.2 THE NULL HYPOTHESIS

Statistical analysis is concerned not only with summarising data but also with investigating relationships. An investigator conducting a study usually has a theory in mind; for example, patients with diabetes have raised blood pressure, or oral contraceptives may cause breast cancer. This theory is known as the *study hypothesis*. However, it is impossible to prove most hypotheses; one can always think of circumstances which have not yet arisen under which it may or may not hold. Thus one might hold a theory that all Chinese children have black hair. Unfortunately, having observed 1000 or even 1 000 000 Chinese children and checked that they all have black hair, would not have proved the hypothesis. On the other hand, if only one fair-haired Chinese child is seen, the theory is disproved. Thus there is a simpler logical setting for disproving hypotheses than for proving them. The converse of the study hypothesis is the *null hypothesis*. Examples are: diabetic patients do not have raised blood pressure, or oral contraceptives do not cause breast cancer. Such a hypothesis is usually phrased in the negative and that is why it is termed null.

Example

Suppose a randomised clinical trial is being conducted to compare two drugs for the treatment of hypertension. In a group of 100 hypertensive patients, half are allocated to receive drug A and half drug B. An appropriate measure of efficacy is determined to be the systolic blood pressure reading (mmHg) after three months of drug use. Further suppose such measurements can be assumed to follow a Normal distribution. The results from the 100 patients are expressed using the group means and standard deviations (SD) as follows:

$$n_A = 50, \ \bar{x}_A = 115, \ SD(x_A) = s_A = 9.9$$

$$n_B = 50, \ \bar{x}_B = 105, \ SD(x_B) = s_B = 10.0$$

Thus $\bar{x}_A = 115$ and $\bar{x}_B = 105$ estimate the two population means μ_A and μ_B respectively. In the context of a clinical trial the population usually refers to those patients, present and future, who have the disease and for whom it would be appropriate to treat with either drug A or B. Now if both drugs are equally effective μ_A equals μ_B and the differences between $\bar{x}_A$ and $\bar{x}_B$ are only chance differences. After all, subjects will differ between themselves, so we would not be surprised if differences between $\bar{x}_A$ and $\bar{x}_B$ are observed, even if the drugs are identical in their activity. The statistical problem is: When can it be concluded that the difference between $\bar{x}_A$ and $\bar{x}_B$ is of sufficient magnitude to suspect that μ_A is not equal to μ_B?

The null hypothesis states that $\mu_A = \mu_B$ and this can be alternatively expressed as $\mu_A - \mu_B = 0$. The problem is to decide if the observations, as expressed by the sample means and corresponding SDs, appear consistent with this hypothesis. Clearly if $\bar{x}_A = \bar{x}_B$ we would be reasonably convinced that $\mu_A = \mu_B$. But what of the actual results given above? To help decide it is necessary to first calculate $\bar{d} = \bar{x}_A - \bar{x}_B = 115 - 105 = 10$ mmHg and also calculate the corresponding standard deviation, $SD(\bar{d})$, which is again usually termed the standard error.

It turns out that

$$SD(\bar{d}) = \sqrt{[SD(\bar{x}_A)^2 + SD(\bar{x}_B)^2]},$$

$$= \sqrt{\left[\frac{s_A{}^2}{n_A} + \frac{s_B{}^2}{n_B} \right]}$$

$$= \sqrt{\left[\frac{9.9^2}{50} + \frac{10.0^2}{50} \right]}$$

$$= 1.99 \text{ mmHg}$$

Now, if indeed the two populations of systolic blood pressure values can be assumed to have approximately Normal distributions, in the two groups, then $\bar{d}$ will also have a Normal distribution. This distribution will have its own mean $\delta = \mu_A - \mu_B$ and standard deviation σ_δ, which are estimated by $\bar{d}$ and $SD(\bar{d})$ respectively. One can even go one step further, if samples are large enough, and state that the ratio $\bar{d}/SD(\bar{d})$ will have a Normal distribution with mean δ and a standard deviation of unity. If the null hypothesis were true, this distribution would have mean $\delta = 0$. However, the observed values are $\bar{d} = 10\,\text{mmHg}$ with $SD(\bar{d}) = 1.99$ and therefore a ratio of mean to standard deviation of 10/1.99 or approximately 5 standard deviations from the null hypothesis mean of zero. This is a very extreme observation and very unlikely to arise by chance since 95% of observations sampled from a Normal distribution with specified mean and standard deviation will be within 1.96 standard deviations of its centre. A value of δ greater than zero seems very plausible. It therefore seems very unlikely that the measurements come from a Normal distribution whose mean is in fact $\delta = \mu_A - \mu_B = 0$. There is strong evidence that μ_A and μ_B differ perhaps by a substantial amount. As a consequence the notion of equality of effect of the two drugs suggested by the null hypothesis is rejected. The conclusion is that drug B results in lower systolic blood pressures in patients with hypertension than does drug A.

The next step is to calculate a confidence interval for δ, the true difference between μ_A and μ_B, in a similar way to confidence intervals described in Chapter 5. A 95% confidence interval is given by

$$\bar{d} - 1.96 \times SD(\bar{d}) \qquad \text{to} \qquad \bar{d} + 1.96 \times SD(\bar{d})$$

The corresponding calculations give a 95% confidence interval for δ of 6.1 to 13.9 mmHg.

The method of analysis used for comparing the mean blood pressure in two groups can be utilised for the comparison of two proportions with minor changes. Thus the population proportions of success, π_A and π_B, replace the population means μ_A and μ_B. Similarly the sample statistics p_A, p_B replace $\bar{x}_A$ and $\bar{x}_B$. Again,

$$\bar{d} = p_A - p_B$$

while

$$SD(\bar{d}) = \sqrt{\left[\frac{p_A q_A}{n_A} + \frac{p_B q_B}{n_B} \right]}$$

Example from the literature

The results of a clinical trial conducted by Familiari *et al.* (1981) comparing two drugs for the treatment of peptic ulcers are summarised in Table 6.1.

Table 6.1   Percentage of peptic ulcers healed by treatment group

Drug	Healed	Not healed	Total	% healed
A: Pirenzepine	23 (*a*)	7 (*c*)	30 (*m*)	76.67
B: Trithiozine	18 (*b*)	13 (*d*)	31 (*n*)	58.06
Total	41 (*r*)	20 (*s*)	61 (*N*)	

Source: Familiari *et al.* (1981).

In an obvious notation $n_P = 30$, $p_P = a/m = 0.7667$, $n_T = 31$, $p_T = b/n = 0.5806$, from which $\bar{d} = 0.1861$ and $SD(\bar{d}) = 0.1175$. The 95% confidence interval for δ is -0.0442 to 0.4164. Thus although there is an observed 19% advantage of pirenzepine (A) over trithiozine (B) the 95% confidence interval includes the null hypothesis value of zero difference. These data therefore appear consistent both with an advantage of pirenzepine over trithiozine of as much as 42% and an advantage of trithiozine over pirenzepine of 4%! It should be noted that although calculations are taken to a precision of four decimal places in this example, the final difference in proportions (or percentages) and confidence intervals are quoted to two significant figures.

6.3 THE p-VALUE

All the examples so far have used 95% when calculating a confidence interval, but other percentages could have been chosen. In fact the choice of 95% is quite arbitrary although it has now become conventional in the medical literature. A general $100(1-\alpha)\%$ confidence interval can be calculated using

$$\bar{d} - z_\alpha \times SD(\bar{d}) \qquad \text{to} \qquad \bar{d} + z_\alpha \times SD(\bar{d})$$

In this expression z_α is the value, along the axis of a Normal distribution (Table T1), which leaves a total probability of α equally divided in the two tails. In particular, if $\alpha = 0.05$, then $100(1-\alpha)\% = 95\%$, $z_\alpha = 1.96$ and the 95% confidence interval is given as before by

$$\bar{d} - 1.96 \times SD(\bar{d}) \qquad \text{to} \qquad \bar{d} + 1.96 \times SD(\bar{d})$$

In the comparison of the two treatments for peptic ulcer, the expression for the more general confidence interval for δ is

$$0.1861 - (z_\alpha \times 0.1175) \qquad \text{to} \qquad 0.1861 + (z_\alpha \times 0.1175)$$

Suppose that z_α is now chosen in this expression, in such a way that the left-hand or lower limit of the above confidence interval equals zero. That is, it just includes the null hypothesis value of $\delta = \pi_A - \pi_B = 0$. Then the resulting equation is

$$0.1861 - (z_\alpha \times 0.1175) = 0$$

This equation can be rewritten to become

$$z_\alpha = 0.1861/0.1175$$

$$= 1.58$$

We can now examine Table T1 to find an α such that $z_\alpha = 1.58$. This determines α to be 0.11 and $100(1-\alpha)\%$ to be 89%. Thus an 89% confidence interval for δ is

$$0.1861 - (1.58 \times 0.1175) \qquad \text{to} \qquad 0.1861 + (1.58 \times 0.1175)$$

or 0 to 0.37. This interval just includes the null hypothesis value of zero difference as required. The value of α so calculated is termed the *p-value*. The *p*-value is the probability of obtaining the observed difference, or a value more extreme, if the null hypothesis is true.

Example

The mean change in blood pressure after treatment in 36 patients with hypertension is 5.0 mmHg with standard deviation 15.0 mmHg. Such data may arise when the subject serves as his or her own control. For example, the blood pressure may be recorded before commencement of treatment and then after one week of treatment.

If, the change in blood pressure, d, was calculated for each patient and if the null hypothesis is true that there is no effect of treatment on blood pressure, then the mean of the 36 d's should be close to zero. The d's are termed the *paired differences* and are the basic observations of interest. Thus $\bar{d} = \Sigma d_i/n = 5.0$ and $SD(d) = \sqrt{\Sigma(d_i - \bar{d})^2/(n-1)} = 15.0$. This gives $SD(\bar{d}) = SD(d)/\sqrt{(n)} = 2.5$ and $z = 5.0/2.5 = 2.0$. The *p*-value is obtained using Table T1 with $z = 2.0$, giving $p = 0.046$.

A statistical *significance test* considers this *p*-value. If it is small, conventionally less than 0.05, the null hypothesis is rejected as implausible. If $p > 0.05$ this is often taken as suggesting that insufficient information is available to discount the null hypothesis.

Example from the literature

Frazer, Sutherst and Holland (1987) give the mean and SD of the severity of symptoms of incontinence determined by a visual analogue scale in women patients. The 58 with genuine stress incontinence had a mean score of 49 mm (SD = 23) and those 26 patients with detrusor instability a mean score of 64 mm (SD = 23).

An appropriate null hypothesis is that the incontinence score is unrelated to the diagnosis of the patients. From the above summary, $\bar{d} = 64 - 49 = 15$ mm, and

$$SD(\bar{d}) = \sqrt{\left[\frac{23^2}{26} + \frac{23^2}{58}\right]} = 5.43$$

The corresponding 95% confidence interval for δ is 4.4 to 25.6 mm. A formal significance test gives $z = 15/5.43 = 2.76$ and use of Table T1 gives $p = 0.0058$. This is much smaller than 0.05 and so we would formally reject the null hypothesis of equal means for the two 'populations' of patients.

6.4 STATISTICAL INFERENCE

Hypothesis testing is a method of choosing between the null hypothesis and an alternative hypothesis. The calculation of the *p*-value is an important part of the procedure. Given a study with a single outcome measure and a statistical test, hypothesis testing can be summarised in three steps:

(1) Choose the significance level, α, of the test.
(2) Conduct the study, observe the outcome and compute the p-value.
(3) If the p-value is smaller than α reject the null hypothesis in favour of the alternative hypothesis; if not, do not reject the null hypothesis, and view it as 'not yet disproven'.

The term *statistically significant* pervades the published medical literature. It is a common mistake to state that it is the probability that the null hypothesis is true. It is not, since the null hypothesis is either true or it is false. The null hypothesis is not, therefore, 'true' or 'false' with a certain probability. However, the p-value can be thought of as a measure of the strength of the belief in the null hypothesis. For example, in the hypothetical problem discussed concerning the treatment of hypertension in 36 patients, $p = 0.046$ and is less than 0.05 and so we might be led to (just) reject the null hypothesis. However, the 95% confidence interval calculated in the usual way is 0.1 to 9.9 mmHg, and almost covers the null hypothesis difference of zero. We may be (and rightly so) a little cautious therefore in our rejection of the null hypothesis. In contrast, for the data concerned with incontinence we would be very confident about rejecting the null hypothesis. Whenever a significance test is used, the corresponding report should quote, if possible, the exact p-value to a sensible number of significant figures together with the value of the corresponding test statistic. Thus, in this example, the results section of the paper describing the study would contain a comment on the actual difference observed, followed by, as a minimum, $z = 2.0$, $p = 0.046$. Merely reporting, whichever appropriate, $p < 0.05$ or worse, $p > 0.05$ or $p =$ NS meaning 'not statistically significant', is not acceptable. The statistical guidelines for contributors to medical journals prepared by Altman *et al.* (1983) and reprinted in Gardner and Altman (1989), discuss presentation of the results of significance tests in some detail and this is also discussed in Chapter 10.

6.5 SMALL SAMPLES OF CONTINUOUS DATA

(a) Student's *t*-distribution

So far the discussion in this chapter has implicitly made two assumptions. The first is that the variable under consideration follows an approximately Normal distribution and the second is that samples from the respective population have always been relatively large. However, it is intuitively obvious that with small samples one can make less precise statements about population parameters than one can with large samples. Thus it is necessary to recognise that if samples are small, $\bar{x}$ and s will not always be necessarily close to μ and σ respectively. How does the sample size influence the calculations? In one way sample size is taken already into account through the calculation of the standard deviation of the mean, $SD(\bar{x})$, when dividing by $\sqrt{n}$, the square root of the sample size. In small samples, however, values of s very far from σ will not be uncommon, and one consequence is that although $\bar{d}$ will still have a Normal distribution, it can no longer be assumed the ratio $\bar{d}/SD(\bar{d})$ will.

As a consequence it is necessary to modify the calculation of both the p-value and a confidence interval. To do this the ratio is relabelled as t rather than z to avoid confusion. For the confidence interval z_α is replaced by t_α, in the expression given for a confidence interval in Section 6.3, to obtain

$$\bar{d} - t_\alpha \times \mathrm{SD}(\bar{d}) \qquad \text{to} \qquad \bar{d} + t_\alpha \times \mathrm{SD}(\bar{d})$$

The ratio $\bar{d}/\mathrm{SD}(\bar{d})$ is then known as *Student's t-statistic* and under the null hypothesis is assumed to be distributed as *Student's t-distribution*.

In the expression for the confidence interval the particular value for t_α depends not only on α but also on the number of *degrees of freedom*, df, on which σ is estimated. Table T2 gives some values of t_α for different values of df and α. Examination of the bottom row of Table T2 shows that with df $= \infty$, that is with very large degrees of freedom, the same value for t_α is obtained as for z_α in Table T1 for each value of α. However, the values of t_α get larger as the df get smaller. This reflects the increasing uncertainty concerning the estimate of σ as sample sizes get smaller.

Example from the literature

The results of a study by Myers *et al.* (1987) give the serum-P levels in 6 subjects before and 2 hours after vaginal administration of a 400-mg P suppository are summarised in Table 6.2.

Table 6.2 Serum-P levels in six subjects before and after administration of a 400-mg P suppository

Subject	Serum-P (ng/dl)			$\log_e$(serum-P)		
	0 hrs	2 hrs	Difference	0 hrs	2 hrs	Difference
1	321	1176	855	5.77	7.07	1.30
2	1000	2174	1174	6.91	7.68	0.77
3	1520	1822	302	7.33	7.51	0.18
4	390	1098	708	5.97	7.00	1.03
5	40	163	123	3.69	5.09	1.40
6	12	87	75	2.48	4.46	1.98
Mean	547.2	1086.7	539.5	5.358	6.468	1.110
SD	595.1	846.6	441.9	1.892	1.351	0.611
Median	355.5	1137.0	505.0	5.800	7.035	1.165

Source: Myers *et al.* (1987).

It is clear from examining the serum-P levels at both zero and 2 hours that the distributions appear skew, although for so few values it is not possible to plot a histogram. A quick check of skewness is to calculate the mean and median of the data values. For the baseline serum-P levels the mean is 547.2 and the median 355.5 ng/dl. If a distribution is symmetric then the population mean and median would coincide in value. This is clearly not the case here. On the logarithmic scale, however the mean is 5.36 and the median 5.87 and are relatively close. A similar effect is seen with the 2-hour data. This suggests that the logarithm of the data may be a scale on which one could assume Normal distributions are appropriate. This could be verified using a Normal probability plot as described in Appendix A16.

Now since each subject is investigated before and after insertion of the vaginal suppository, it is natural to calculate the difference between successive values within each woman, and regard these as the basic 6 observations. It is a common mistake to assume in such cases that because the basic observations appear not to have Normal distributions then the methods described here do not apply. It is the before-and-after differences that have to be checked for the assumption of a Normal distribution and not the zero and 2-hour serum values themselves (see Section 6.10 for further discussion).

In fact, the differences calculated from the original (untransformed) scale do not appear to have a Normal distribution since the mean and median are not very close. However, on the logarithmic scale the mean difference $\bar{d} = 1.110$ while the median difference is 1.165. This is very close to the mean and hence it is not unreasonable to assume that these differences have an approximately Normal distribution. We therefore use $SD(d) = 0.611$, and hence $SD(\bar{d}) = 0.611/\sqrt{6} = 0.249$. This is a small study and so we need to use the confidence interval with t_α in place of z_α. In this example, the data are paired and the degrees of freedom are therefore one less than the number of patients in the study, that is $df = n - 1$. Hence, $df = 6 - 1 = 5$ and the 95% confidence interval for the mean difference will be

$$1.110 - (t_{0.05} \times 0.249) \quad \text{to} \quad 1.110 + (t_{0.05} \times 0.249)$$

From Table T2 with $df = 5$, $t_{0.05} = 2.571$, giving the confidence interval as 0.47 to 1.75.

The statistic $\bar{d}$ and the corresponding confidence interval are not easy to interpret as we have used the logarithmic scale in the calculations. However, if we now take the antilogarithm of $\bar{d}$ we obtain 3.03 which now represents an average ratio of the 2-hour to zero-hour readings. In fact this can be arrived at without the use of logarithms at all. First calculate the ratio for each subject, multiply the six ratios together and then take the sixth root. This process gives $\bar{x}_G = 3.03$. Such an average is termed a *geometric* mean.

If we take the antilogarithm of the respective confidence limits of 0.47 and 1.75 we obtain a 95% confidence interval for the population ratio of 2-hour to zero-hour serum-P levels of 1.6 to 5.8. The null hypothesis, of course, implies a difference in population means of zero which in turn implies a ratio of unity.

(b) Pooling standard deviations

When discussing the comparison of the two populations with means μ_A and μ_B it was stated that

$$SD(\bar{d}) = \sqrt{\left[\frac{s_A^2}{n_A} + \frac{s_B^2}{n_B}\right]}$$

where $\bar{d} = \bar{x}_A - \bar{x}_B$ and s_A and s_B are estimates of the population standard deviations σ_A and σ_B. With small samples the first step is often to assume that $\sigma_A = \sigma_B$ (although methods are available for checking if this is reasonable). It was a coincidence that s_A

and s_B were both equal to 23 mm in the example in Section 6.3 taken from Frazer *et al*. (1987). If the populations do have the same standard deviation then s_A and s_B both estimate the same quantity σ. It can be shown that the best estimate of σ is s_P, which is calculated from a weighted average of the squares of s_A and s_B, using the expression given in Appendix A4. The appropriate degrees of freedom are then given by df = $(n_A - 1) + (n_B - 1)$.

Using s_P in place of s_A and s_B gives

$$SD(\bar{d}) = \sqrt{\left[\frac{s_P^2}{n_A} + \frac{s_P^2}{n_B}\right]}$$

Example from the literature

Larochelle *et al*. (1987) give the plasma atrial natriuretic factor concentration in blood taken from the aorta in 7 patients with essential hypertension as 25.0 ng/l (SE = 6.0) and in 8 patients with renovascular hypertension as 46.5 ng/l (SE = 10.2).

This gives $\bar{d} = 46.5 - 25.0 = 21.5$ ng/l. Now using the fact that $SE(\bar{x}) = SD(x)/\sqrt{n}$, we can back calculate the standard deviations of the two groups of patients as 15.9 and 28.8 ng/l respectively. This leads to the pooled estimate of the standard deviation as

$$s_P = \sqrt{([6 \times 15.9^2 + 7 \times 28.8^2]/[6 + 7])}$$

$$= 23.7$$

and

$$SD(\bar{d}) = \sqrt{\left[\frac{23.7^2}{7} + \frac{23.7^2}{8}\right]} = 12.3$$

Using Table T2 with $\alpha = 0.05$ and df = 6 + 7 = 13 gives $t_{0.05} = 2.160$. Thus the 95% confidence interval for δ becomes

$$21.5 - (2.160 \times 12.3) \quad \text{to} \quad 21.5 + (2.160 \times 12.3)$$

or -5.1 to 48.1 ng/l

This confidence interval includes the null hypothesis value of zero difference between diagnostic groups. However, there is considerable uncertainty surrounding the true difference, δ, as the confidence interval is so wide.

As already indicated, in small samples we also need to modify the corresponding significance tests. To do this we refer t, the ratio of the statistic to its standard deviation, to Table T2 rather than Table T1. In this example $t = 21.5/12.3 = 1.75$, df= 13 and use of Table T2 gives $p \approx 0.1$. This is not therefore formally statistically significant at the 5% level.

If s_A and s_B cannot be assumed to estimate a common value, special steps have to be taken. In some situations a transformation may result in approximately equal standard deviations in the two groups. In other situations the large-sample expression is retained for $SD(\bar{d})$ but the df are taken as a weighted mean of $(n_A - 1)$ and $(n_B - 1)$. Details can be found in, for example, Armitage and Berry (1987).

6.6 THE χ^2 TEST

(a) 2×2 contingency tables

To illustrate how the test for a comparison of proportions can be modified to cover the situation of small samples it is useful to refer to Table 6.1, which summarises the results of the peptic ulcer study of Familiari *et al.* (1981) and to use the notation given in the table. This gives $a = 23$, $b = 18$, $c = 7$ and $d = 13$.

The first step is to obtain a pooled estimate of the standard deviation of the difference in proportions in a similar way to when comparing two means. Now if the null hypothesis is true p_A and p_B both estimate a common parameter π, which is best estimated by $p = r/N = 41/61 = 0.6721$.

Readers should note there is a possibility of some confusion here, as p is used as the overall proportion of treatment successes and not the p-value itself. This multiple usage of p is common throughout the medical literature.

The corresponding standard deviation is then calculated by replacing both p_A and p_B by p so that

$$SD(p_A - p_B) = \sqrt{\left[\frac{pq}{m} + \frac{pq}{n}\right]}$$

where $q = 1 - p$. Thus

$$SD(p_A - p_B) = \sqrt{[pq(1/m + 1/n)]}$$

$$= \sqrt{[0.6721 \times 0.3279 (1/30 + 1/31)]}$$

$$= 0.1202$$

For a significance test we now calculate

$$z = (p_A - p_B)/SD(p_A - p_B) = 0.1175/0.1202 = 1.548$$

This calculation can be expressed in terms of the algebraic notation of the 2×2 contingency table (Table 6.1). It turns out that z^2, (and by convention we denote this by χ^2 rather than z^2), is exactly

$$\chi^2 = \frac{N(ad - bc)^2}{mnrs}$$

This test is termed the χ^2 or chi-squared test. This leads to $\chi^2 = 2.3940$, which is equal to the square of 1.548 except for a small rounding error.

In examples which have a small number of subjects it is only necessary to modify the expression for χ^2 in the following manner

$$\chi_c^2 = \frac{N\{|ad - bc| - \frac{1}{2}N\}^2}{mnrs}$$

The notation of the vertical lines means calculate $ad - bc$ but, whatever the sign of the result, treat it as positive. The subtraction of $\frac{1}{2}N$ causes χ_c^2 to be smaller than χ^2. The device of reduction in the numerator by $\frac{1}{2}N$ is usually referred to as *Yates' correction for continuity*. For the peptic ulcer example $\chi_c^2 = 1.62$.

Special tables have been constructed which allow the statistical significance of χ^2, or χ_c^2, to be assessed directly. Thus rather than taking the square root of χ_c^2 and referring to Table T1 we can refer to the first row of Table T3 with df = 1. Here we find with $\alpha = 0.2$ a tabular entry of 1.64, which is close to the calculated $\chi_c^2 = 1.62$. Thus the significance level or *p*-value is approximately 0.2. It should be added that the device of taking the square root of χ^2 and referring to Table T1 is only valid in the case when the df = 1. In all other situations Table T3 has to be used.

An alternative method of calculating the chi-squared test, using *expected* counts under the null hypothesis, is given in Appendix A6. Where the expected counts are low (less than 5 is the usual recommendation) it is better to use *Fisher's exact test* described in Appendix A7 to determine the *p*-value.

(b) Contingency tables with more than two rows or columns

Example from the literature

Nichols *et al.* (1986) give the compliance with screening for colorectal cancer by means of the haemoccult test with respect to the method of invitation to screening. A summary of some of their results is given in Table 6.3.

The overall compliance rate is $7545/17824 = 0.423$, or 42.3%. If compliance is not influenced by the method of invitation then the expected number of subjects to comply would be 42.3% of each invitation group. Thus on this basis, of the 6261 subjects

Table 6.3 Compliance with screening by invitation group (expected values in brackets)

Method of invitation	Number of subjects			% Complied
	Complied	Did not comply	Total	
Letter + test	3108 (3441.5)	5028 (4694.5)	8136	38.2
Letter	2468 (2648.4)	3793 (3612.6)	6261	39.4
Consultation	1969 (1449.6)	1458 (1977.4)	3427	57.5
	7545	10279	17824	42.3

Source: Nichols *et al.* (1986).

receiving an invitation by letter only, one would expect $0.423 \times 6261 = 2648.4$ to comply with screening. The expected number of subjects, E, for each entry in the above table is indicated by the bracketed figure.

The general expression for χ^2 is

$$\chi^2 = \sum \frac{(O - E)^2}{E}$$

where O are the observed values and the summation extends over all the cells of the contingency tables. In this case there are 6 cells and $\chi^2 = 399.84$.

This value is then referred to Table T3 with df$= (r - 1)(c - 1)$ where r and c are the number of rows (here 3) and columns (here 2) of the contingency table, hence df $= 2$. It is clear that even for $\alpha = 0.001$ the tabulation value of 13.82 is much less than $\chi^2 = 399.84$ and so $p < 0.001$. Thus there is a highly statistically significant difference in compliance rates between methods of invitation. It is clear that this comes from the greater compliance rate from the consultation group. A further example is given in Appendix A8.

An important class of tests occurs when one of the classifying variables is ordered and the other has only two levels. We can then use the more powerful *chi-squared test for trend* described in Appendix A8.

6.7 PAIRED COMPARISONS IN CONTINGENCY TABLES

Just as for continuous data, a special analysis is required if paired or matched data are involved. Paired data often arise from cross-over clinical trials and matched-pair case-control studies.

Example from the literature

Consider the study of testicular cancer by Brown, Pottern and Hoover (1987), referred to in Section 2.7. They conducted a matched case-control study, and one of the questions asked of both cases and controls was whether or not their testes were descended at birth. Part of the results of their study is given in Table 6.4.

Table 6.4   Results of a matched case-control study

| | | Controls | | |
		Undescended testes (exposed)	No undescended testes (not exposed)	Total
Cases	Undescended testes	4(*e*)	11(*f*)	15
	No undescended testes	3(*g*)	241(*h*)	244
Total		7	252	261

Source: Brown *et al.* (1987).

Consider the following four case-control pairs:

Pair 1 Both with undescended testes
Pair 2 Both with descended testes
Pair 3 Case with undescended testes, control with descended testes
Pair 4 Case with descended tests, control with undescended testes

If all matched pairs were like pairs 1 and 2 we would be unable to answer the question: 'Do undescended testes result in a greater risk of testicular cancer?' It is only the discordant pairs 3 and 4 that provide relevant information in that cases and controls differ in their response. It is important to note that it is only the numbers of pairs 3 and 4 that influence the test of hypothesis, and it does not matter how many matched pairs of type 1 or 2 there are. If there were many more matched pairs like pair 3 than pair 4 we would have evidence against the null hypothesis, and answer the above question in the affirmative. If there were about the same number of matched pairs like pair 3 and pair 4, we would answer the above question in the negative. If there were many more matched pairs like pair 4 than pair 3, we would have evidence that undescended testes exert a protective effect.

In this example the appropriate null hypothesis is that the expected values of f and g will be equal. Given that there are $f + g$ discordant pairs, we would expect half to be pair 3 (cases exposed, controls not). Thus $O_1 = f$ while $E_1 = (f + g)/2$ and $O_2 = g$ while $E_2 = (f + g)/2$. A χ^2 test using the general expression of Section 6.6 would be

$$\chi^2 = \frac{(O_1 - E_1)^2}{E_1} + \frac{(O_2 - E_2)^2}{E_2}$$

$$= \frac{(f - g)^2}{f + g}$$

This test statistic is called McNemar's test. It may be adjusted for small values of either f or g, to

$$\chi_M^2 = \frac{(|f - g| - 1)^2}{(f + g)}$$

The correction of -1 makes little difference to the calculations in large samples. For the data of Brown *et al*, we have

$$\chi_M^2 = \frac{(|11 - 3| - 1)^2}{(11 + 3)} = 3.5$$

We compare this with the tabulated values of χ^2 with df = 1 in Table T3. This indicates that $p \approx 0.05$. In fact, more exact calculations by taking the square root of 3.5 and referring to Table T1 give $p = 0.06$ and so we do not have strong evidence to reject the null hypothesis. A further example of McNemar's test is given in Appendix A9. The exact test for paired data, equivalent to Fisher's exact test for unpaired data, is also described there.

6.8 WHEN IS 'LARGE' LARGE ENOUGH?

In the case of continuous variables it has been indicated that if samples are small it is usual to use the t-distribution rather than the Normal distribution when calculating the final p-value or confidence interval. A glance at any column of Table T2 shows that as the degrees of freedom, df, get larger the corresponding value of t for a given α gets closer and closer to the corresponding z value in the Normal distribution of Table T1, which are also given in Table T2 along the row with infinite degrees of freedom. Thus an investigator will always be on the 'safe side' by assuming all samples are small. Similar considerations apply to the χ^2 test for 2×2 contingency tables. As a guide therefore it is sensible to use t and χ_c^2 as a matter of routine. As already stated, the χ_c^2 test is an approximation to what is known as *Fisher's exact test*. The usual rule is that Fisher's exact test should be used if any of the expected values are less than 5. However, the χ^2 test with continuity correction will lead to a good approximation to the p-value obtained from the Fisher exact test provided all the expected values are greater than unity.

There is no simple procedure for contingency tables with more than two rows or columns and small numbers.

6.9 STATISTICAL POWER

If one rejects the null hypothesis when it is in fact true, then one makes what is known as a *Type I error*. The significance level α is the probability of making a Type I error when the null hypothesis is true. However, there is another error one can make; that is not rejecting the null hypothesis when it is in fact false. This is known as the *Type II error*, and the probability of making a Type II error is designated β. The *power* of the study equals $1 - \beta$ and is the probability of rejecting the null hypothesis when it is false. In general, larger studies are more powerful, in that they have greater ability to reject the null hypothesis.

Example from the literature

In a randomised trial of 1239 patients, Elwood and Sweetnam (1979) discovered the mortality after a non-fatal myocardial infarction to be 8.0% in a group given aspirin and 10.7% in a group given placebo. The difference 2.7% has 95% confidence interval -0.5% to 6.0%.

Based on this result, a reader might conclude that there was little evidence for an effect of aspirin on mortality after myocardial infarction. However, shortly after this another study was published, the Persantine–Aspirin Reinfarction Study (1980). This showed 9.2% mortality in the aspirin group, and 11.5% in the placebo, a difference of 2.3%, which is less than that of Elwood and Sweetnam. However, the sample size was 6292 and the 95% confidence interval 0.8% to 3.8%. The larger study had greater power, and so achieved narrower confidence intervals.

As an aside, there is a general methodology for combining results from two or more studies. It is usually termed *meta-analysis* or *over-views*. It is beyond the scope of this book, but a useful review is given by Last (1987).

6.10 NON-NORMAL DISTRIBUTIONS

(a) Non-parametric tests

It was indicated above that for continuous variables an underlying Normal distribution is assumed. If this appears not to be the case, even after taking a transformation of the basic variable and working on the new scale, then alternative procedures are available which do not assume Normality. In such situations the paired t-test is replaced by the Wilcoxon signed-rank sum test, and the unpaired test by the Wilcoxon test alternatively described as the Mann–Whitney U test. Details of these tests are given in Appendix A10. These tests remain the same for large or small samples but may be tedious to calculate in the large-sample cases. Special tables are usually required in the small-sample cases. These tests are often termed *distribution-free* or *non-parametric tests*.

(b) Why not always use non-parametric tests?

It can been argued that since non-parametric tests can always be used, why not use them always! The argument has much appeal but can be answered albeit in somewhat technical terms. It turns out that if a non-parametric test is used when the data follow a Normal distribution, then the calculated p-value will always exceed that that would be obtained using the Student t-test. Thus one is less likely to declare a result significant using a non-parametric test than using a parametric test with the same data. This is because the more assumptions one is prepared to make about the data, the more precisely one can investigate hypotheses. In these circumstances the non-parametric test is termed less powerful, although the loss of power is often not very great. The corresponding non-parametric confidence intervals will also be wider and more difficult to calculate, although help with this is provided by Campbell and Gardner (1988).

However, the overwhelming argument against the routine use of non-parametric procedures is that they are not flexible enough. For example, they do not allow for analyses such as multiple regression and the analysis of covariance, which take into account other characteristics of the groups being compared. There is also some misunderstanding about the flexibility of parametric tests. For example, for the data summarised in Table 6.2, it was indicated that a Normal distribution does not seem reasonable for either the 0 or 2 hour readings. However, this does not in itself invalidate the use of Student's t-test as it is only necessary that the variable used for the statistical analysis, in this case a measure of the difference in the two levels for each subject, has an approximately Normal distribution. Bland (1987) gives a useful discussion on the limitations of parametric and non-parametric tests.

6.11 DEGREES OF FREEDOM

The number of degrees of freedom, df, has been discussed in two situations: the first with respect to t-tests and the second with respect to χ^2 tests. In fact the number of degrees of freedom depends on two factors: Firstly the number of groups we wish to compare and secondly the number of parameters we need to estimate to calculate the standard deviation of the contrast of interest. Thus for the χ^2 test for the comparison of two proportions, which is equivalent to a z test in large samples, there are two groups to compare, hence there is 1 degree of freedom for the between-groups comparison. Once the proportion is estimated in each group, a direct estimate of the standard error is $\sqrt{(pq/n)}$, without estimation of an additional parameter. This is because the binomial distribution, for a particular n, is completely determined by p.

In contrast, when comparing two means, whereas there is still 1 degree of freedom for between-groups, there are also degrees of freedom for estimating σ. How the df are calculated depends on the particular problem. For a paired situation df equals the number of subjects minus one; for an unpaired situation it is the total number of subjects minus 2, that is $n-1$ for each group. Thus the t-test has two sets of degrees of freedom attached to it. The first, 1 degree of freedom for between-groups, the second for within-groups. However, since the t-test always concerns the comparison of two groups, the first of these df, is not usually explicitly referred to. The z-test is similar to the t-test but since in this case σ is assumed known then effectively the within-groups df are infinite and these also are not explicitly referred to.

The t-test is generalised to more than two groups by means of a technique termed the *analysis of variance*. For this method there are both between- and within-groups degrees of freedom. The method is applicable in more than two group comparisons, and so we quote both the between-groups and within-groups degrees of freedom, in that order, in every case.

6.12 CONFIDENCE INTERVALS RATHER THAN p-VALUES

Simple statements such as '$p < 0.05$' or '$p = NS$' do not describe the results of a study well, and create an artificial dichotomy between significant and non-significant results. The p-value does not relate to the clinical importance of a finding, and it depends to a large extent on the size of the study. Thus a large study may find small, unimportant, differences that are highly significant and a small study may fail to find important differences. The confidence interval gives an estimate of the precision with which a statistic estimates a population value, which is useful information for the reader. This does not mean that one should not carry out statistical tests and quote p-values, rather that these results should supplement an estimate of an effect and a confidence interval. Many medical journals now require papers to contain confidence intervals where appropriate. A useful book, containing many techniques for estimating confidence intervals in different situations, is that edited by Gardner and Altman (1989).

6.13 POINTS WHEN READING THE LITERATURE

(1) Have clinical importance and statistical significance been confused?
(2) Has the sample size been taken into account when determining the choice of statistical tests, that is, are small-sample tests used when appropriate?
(3) For 2×2 tables, has a continuity corrrection been used in the analysis. If not, why not? If the counts are low, has an exact test been used?

(4) Is it reasonable to assume that the continuous variables have a Normal distribution?
(5) Have paired tests been utilised in the appropriate places?
(6) Have confidence intervals of the main results been quoted?
(7) Is the result biologically or clinically plausible and has the statistical significance of the result been considered in isolation, or have other studies of the same effect been taken into account?

Chapter 7

Correlation and linear regression

Summary

Correlation and linear regression are techniques for dealing with the relationship between two or more continuous variables. In correlation we are looking for a linear association between two variables, and the strength of the association is summarised by the correlation coefficient. This is a dimensionless quantity ranging from -1 to +1. In regression we are looking for a dependence of one variable, the dependent variable on another, the independent variable. The relationship is summarised by a regression equation consisting of a slope and an intercept. The slope represents the amount the dependent variable increases with unit increase in the independent variable, and the intercept represents the value of the dependent variable when the independent variable takes the value zero. In multiple regression we are interested in the simultaneous relationship between one dependent variable and a number of independent variables.

7.1 INTRODUCTION

The appropriate statistic for examining associations between discrete variables is the chi-squared statistic. When the variables are continuous, however, there is much greater scope for exploring a variety of associations.

The simplest question to ask in this situation is: 'Is there a linear association between the variables?' This is the question answered by correlation. Godfrey (1985) gives a large number of examples of the use of correlation in the *New England Journal of Medicine*. As an example, Mountain, Zwillich and Weil (1978) describe an investigation into the association between alveolar oxygen tension and minute ventilation of oxygen.

Where it is believed that one variable is a direct cause of the other, or that if the values of one variable is changed, then as a direct consequence the other variable also changes, then the associations between them should be explored using linear regression rather than by simple correlation. The simplest method of describing a relationship between two continuous variables is by a straight line. In this case one variable changes directly in proportion to the other, and this type of relationship has proved very useful in medical research. An example of the use of regression techniques is given by Loirat *et al.* (1978), who looked at the relation between the renal clearance of creatinine in patients with burns and their age in years. It makes sense to think of age as possibly reducing creatinine clearance, whereas creatinine clearance could hardly influence age! The relationship between the two variables is therefore best explored using regression techniques.

In a review of four volumes of the *New England Journal of Medicine*, Emerson and Colditz (1983) discovered that authors from 12% of the papers used correlation and 8% simple linear regression techniques. It is clear that an understanding of correlation and linear regression is important for an understanding of many medical papers.

Example from the literature

Campbell, Elwood, Mackean and Waters (1985) invited women, in a pre-defined geographical area, to have their haemoglobin (Hb) level and packed cell volume (PCV) measured. They were also asked their age, and whether or not they had experienced the menopause. The response rate to the invitation was about 90%. Results from a random sample of 20 women from the group are given in Table 7.1 and we use these data to illustrate the ideas underlying correlation and linear regression.

Table 7.1 Haemoglobin level (Hb), packed cell volume (PCV), age and menopausal status in a group of 20 women

Subject number	Hb (g/dl)	PCV (%)	Age (yrs)	Menopause 1=No 0=Yes
1	11.1	35	20	1
2	10.7	45	22	1
3	12.4	47	25	1
4·	14.0	50	28	1
5	13.1	31	28	1
6	10.5	30	31	1
7	9.6	25	32	1
8	12.5	33	35	1
9	13.5	35	38	1
10	13.9	40	40	1
11	15.1	45	45	0
12	13.9	47	49	1
13	16.2	49	54	0
14	16.3	42	55	0
15	16.8	40	57	0
16	17.1	50	60	0
17	16.6	46	62	0
18	16.9	55	63	0
19	15.7	42	65	0
20	16.5	46	67	0

Source: Part data from Campbell *et al.* (1985).

7.2 CORRELATION

(a) Some facts about the correlation coefficient

In Chapter 4 we described methods of plotting data when associations between two variables are to be explored. In such cases we would like a statistic that summarises the strength of the relationship, in much the same way that the mean and standard deviation summarise the centre and variability of the data.

Example

Consider the scatter diagram in Figure 7.1, which illustrates the relationship between haemoglobin level and packed cell volume in the 20 women of Table 7.1.

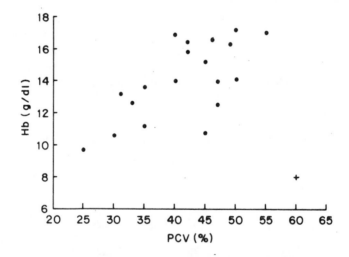

Figure 7.1   Scatter diagram of haemoglobin and packed cell volume in 20 women (part data from Campbell *et al.*, 1985)

In this situation we are not really interested in causation, that is whether a high packed cell volume *causes* a high haemoglobin level, but rather: Is a high packed cell volume *associated* with a high haemoglobin level? The sample *correlation coefficient*, r, enables us not only to summarise the strength of the relationship but also to test the hypothesis that the population correlation coefficient p is zero. That is whether an apparent association between the variables could have arisen by chance. The formula for calculating the correlation coefficient and testing its significance is given in Appendix A11.

When the correlation coefficient is based on the original observations it is known as the Pearson correlation coefficient. When it is calculated from the ranks of the data it is known as the Spearman rank correlation coefficient.

The correlation coefficient is a dimensionless quantity ranging from -1 to $+1$. A positive correlation is one in which both variables increase together. A negative correlation is one in which one variable increases as the other decreases. When variables are exactly linearly related, then the correlation coefficient either equals $+1$ or -1. Values for different strengths of association are shown in Figure 7.2.

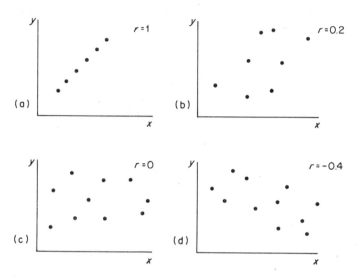

Figure 7.2   Scatter plot showing data sets with different correlations: (a) strong positive, (b) weak positive, (c) uncorrelated and (d) weak negative

The correlation coefficient is unaffected by the units of measurement. Thus, if assessing the strength of association between, say, blood pressure and age it does not matter whether blood pressure is measured in mmHg, lb per square inch or kPa per square cm, as the correlation coefficient remains unaffected.

The square of the correlation coefficient gives the proportion of the variation of one variable 'explained' by the other. Thus a correlation coefficient of 0.9 means that $0.9^2 = 0.81$ or about 80% of the variation in one variable can be accounted for by the other.

(b)   When not to use the correlation coefficient

To determine whether the correlation coefficient is an appropriate measure of association, a first step should always be to look at a plot of the data. The situations where it might be inappropriate to use the correlation coefficient are detailed below.

(i) The correlation coefficient should not be used if the relationship is non-linear. Figure 7.3(a) shows a situation in which y is related to x by means of the equation $y = a + bx + cx^2$. In this case it is possible to predict y exactly for each value of x. There is therefore a perfect association between x and y. However, it turns out that r is not equal to one. This is because the expression for y involves an x^2 term, or what is known as a quadratic term, and so the relationship is *non-linear* as is clear from the figure. Figure 7.3(b) shows a situation in which y is also clearly strongly associated with x and yet the correlation coefficient is zero. Such an example may arise if y represented overall mortality of a population and x some measure of obesity. Very thin and very fat people have higher mortality than people with average weight for their height.

In the situations depicted by both Figure 7.3(a) and (b) there is clearly a close relationship between y and x, but it is not linear. In situations such as these, one should abandon trying to find a single summary statistic of the relationship, and instead try to find a model for it, perhaps using multiple regression which is discussed in Section 7.3.

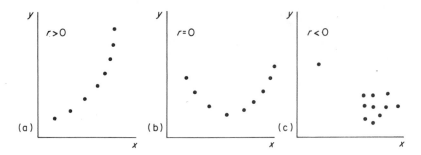

Figure 7.3 Examples where use of the correlation coefficient is inappropriate

(ii) The correlation coefficient should be used with caution in the presence of outliers. For example, Figure 7.3c shows a situation in which one observation is well outside the main body of the data. This observation has a great deal of influence on the estimated value of the correlation coefficient. Since it is so extreme it is possible that this observation in fact comes from a different population from the others. Such an observation may arise in a study of blood loss and its relation to initial haemoglobin level following insertion of an IUD. The outlier might be one woman who happens to have a disease that causes heavy blood loss and also renders her anaemic. If she is excluded from the data set, the correlation coefficient becomes close to zero for the remainder.

(iii) The correlation coefficient should be used with caution when the variables are measured over more than one distinct group, for example patients with a disease and healthy controls. Such studies may result in two clusters of points with zero correlation and produce the same effect as the outlier in Figure 7.3c.

(iv) The correlation coefficient should not be used in situations where one of the variables is determined in advance. For example, if one was measuring responses to different doses of a drug, one would not summarise the relationship with a correlation coefficient. It can be shown that the choice of the particular drug dose levels used by the experimenter will result in different correlation coefficients, even though the underlying dose–response relationship is fixed (see also Section 7.2(a) below).

(c) Tests of significance

Having plotted the data, and established that it is plausible the two variables are associated linearly, we have to decide whether the observed correlation could have arisen by chance, since even if there were no association between the variables, the correlation coefficient is extremely unlikely to be exactly zero. The test of significance is described in Appendix A11.

Example

For the data from Figure 7.1, the correlation between haemoglobin and packed cell volume is found to be $r = 0.67$.

With the number of observations $n = 20$ the test yields a t-statistic of 3.86 with 18 degrees of freedom. From Table T2, $t_{0.01} = 2.878$, hence $p < 0.01$. Thus the relationship can be summarised by saying there is a correlation of 0.67, and the probability of such a correlation, or one more extreme, arising by chance when there is in fact no relation is less than 1 in 100. Thus we reject the null hypothesis and accept that Hb and PCV are associated.

(d) Assumptions underlying the test of significance

The assumption underlying the test of significance is that both variables are random samples from Normal distributions. This is to be contrasted with the assumptions underlying tests of significance in linear regression, to be discussed later. Outlying points, away from the main body of the data, suggest the variable may not have a Normal distribution and hence invalidate the test of significance. In this case, it may be better to replace the observations by their ranks and use the Spearman rank correlation coefficient.

Example

Consider an additional subject for Table 7.1, with a haemoglobin level of 8g/dl and a PCV of 60%, shown by a '+' in Figure 7.1.

As one can see from Figure 7.1, such a woman is well outside the main body of the data. The correlation coefficient is now reduced to 0.29, and the test of significance becomes $t = 1.32$, df = 19 and use of Table T2 gives $p > 0.10$, which is no longer statistically significant.

For the 20 women of Table 7.1 the corresponding Spearman rank correlation coefficient without the outlying point is $r = 0.63$, df = 18 and $p < 0.01$. Including the outlying point reduces r to 0.41, with df=19 and $p < 0.05$. Thus, the change is not as great as for the Pearson correlation coefficient. The overall effect of the additional point is to reduce the correlation, and to render the statistical test less significant.

7.3 REGRESSION

(a) The regression line

When considering the correlation between two variables y and x we are usually not interested in whether y predicts x or vice versa. In *regression*, however, we assume that a change in x will lead directly to a change in y, and that essentially x *causes* y. Usually, it would not be logical to believe that y caused x. The y variable is termed the *dependent* variable and the x variable the *independent* variable. It is conventional to plot the dependent variable on the vertical or y-axis and the independent variable on the horizontal or x-axis.

Example

The data from Table 7.1 on age and haemoglobin level are plotted in Figure 7.4.

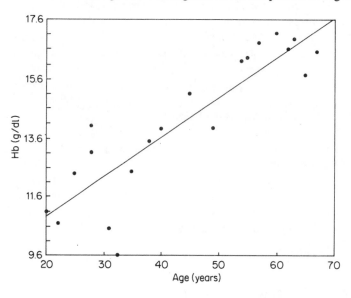

Figure 7.4   Scatter plot of haemoglobin and age in 20 women together with the corresponding regression line

It is logical to believe that increasing age may affect haemoglobin level, and not the other way around.

The equation $y = \alpha + \beta x$ is called the *regression equation*, where α is the *intercept*, and β is the *regression coefficient*. The regression equation is an example of what is often termed a *model* with which attempts to model or describe the relationship between y and x. On a graph, α is the value of the equation when $x = 0$, and β is the *slope* of the line. When x increases by one unit, y is expected to change by β units. Given a series of n pairs of observations (x_1, y_1), (x_2, y_2), ... , (x_n, y_n), in which we believe that y is linearly related to x, what is the best method of estimating α and β? As in earlier chapters we think of the parameters α and β as characteristics of a population and we require estimates of these parameters calculated from a sample taken from the population. We label these estimates a and b respectively.

If we had estimates for a and b we could predict for each x_i the value of y_i by $Y_i = a + bx_i$. Clearly, we would like to choose a and b so that y_i and Y_i are close and hence make the overall prediction error as small as possible. This can be done by choosing a and b to minimise the sum $\Sigma(y_i - Y_i)^2$. For this reason a and b are called the *least squares estimates* of the *population parameters* α and β. The method of calculation of the least squares estimates for α and β is given in Appendix A12. From the data in Table 7.1 it is found that $a = 8.24$ and $b = 0.134$; the corresponding fitted regression line is shown in Figure 7.4.

As discussed in Chapter 5, sample estimates have an inherent variability, estimated by the standard error which is also given in Appendix A12. To calculate the degrees of freedom associated with the standard error, given n independent pairs of observations, 2 degrees of freedom are removed for the two parameters that have been estimated. Thus there are $n - 2$ degrees of freedom.

(b) Tests of significance and confidence intervals

To test the hypothesis that there is no association between haemoglobin and age, we compare $b/SE(b)$ with a t-statistic with $n - 2$ degrees of freedom.

Example

From Table 7.1, the following result is obtained for the relationship between haemoglobin and age: $b = 0.134$ g/dl/yr, $SE(b) = 0.017$ and df $= 18$.

The interpretation of b is that we expect haemoglobin to increase by 0.134 g/dl for every year of age. The corresponding test for significance is given by calculating $t = 0.134/0.017 = 7.84$. Use of Table T2 with df $= 18$ gives $p < 0.001$.
  A 95% confidence interval for β with $n - 2$ degrees of freedom is given by

$$b - t_{0.05} \times SE(b) \qquad \text{to} \qquad b + t_{0.05} \times SE(b)$$

For this example from Table T2 we can obtain $t_{0.05} = 2.101$ as the 5% value with 18 df. Thus the 95% confidence interval for β is given by

$$0.134 - 2.101 \times 0.017 \qquad \text{to} \qquad 0.134 + 2.101 \times 0.017$$

which is 0.10 to 0.17 g/dl/yr.

(c) Assumptions underlying the test of significance

(i) The relationship is approximately linear. This is most easily verified by plotting y_i against x_i as shown in Figure 7.4. A further plot that can be useful is to plot the *residuals* $R_i = y_i - Y_i$, that is the observed y minus the predicted y, against x_i. If there is any discernible relationship between the residuals and x_i, then it is likely that the relationship between y_i and x_i is not linear.

Example

The plot of the residuals remaining after fitting age to haemoglobin against the dependent variable, age, for the data in Table 7.1 is given in Figure 7.5.
  There is no discernible correlation, so we conclude that the linear regression provides an adequate model with which to describe the data. If the graph had indicated a correlation it would suggest that perhaps some other variable may also be influencing haemoglobin levels in addition to age.

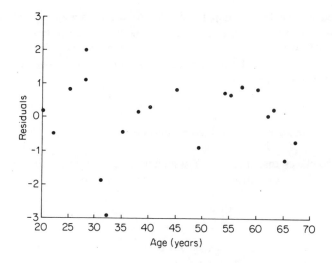

Figure 7.5   A scatter plot of residuals from linear regression against age

(ii) The prediction error is unrelated to the size of the independent variable. It sometimes happens that if a small x is predicting a small y the residual is much smaller than when a large x is predicting a large y. A useful plot to examine if this is the case is of the residuals R_i against the fitted values Y_i. If the residuals appear to get larger with increasing x, then the assumption that they are independent of the value of x clearly cannot hold. If this is the case, then one may attempt to remedy the situation by using a transformation of the y variable and then repeat both the calculation of the regression line and the plots. A useful transformation to try is the logarithmic one.

Example

The plot of the residuals against the fitted values is shown in Figure 7.6.

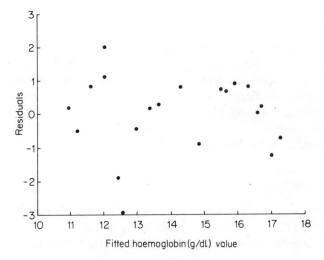

Figure 7.6   A scatter plot of residuals for linear regression against fitted values

There is some evidence in this plot that the scatter of the residuals is actually decreasing with increasing haemoglobin. This would suggest that age is not the only variable to determine haemoglobin levels.

(iii) The residuals about the fitted line are Normally distributed. This does not imply that the y_i's themselves must be Normally distributed, or even that they must be continuous variables. Thus a simple rating scale variable may only take values such as 0, 1, 2, 3 but when related to some x variable by means of linear regression, may give residuals about that line that are Normally distributed. One method of verifying Normality is to plot the histogram of the residuals, with the best fit Normal curve superimposed on it. An example of a best fit Normal curve is given in Figure 5.1. A more efficient way of examining the results is to plot the residuals against their ordered Normal scores or Normal ordinates, as described in Appendix A16. Deviations from linearity indicate lack of Normality.

Example

A scatter plot of the ordered Normal scores is shown in Figure 7.7.

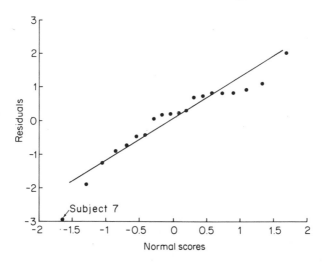

Figure 7.7   A scatter plot of residuals from the linear regression of Figure 7.4 against their ordered Normal scores

It can be seen from Figure 7.7 that the data are plausibly Normally distributed although there is a possibility that the residual corresponding to subject 7 is rather too low to be considered part of the same sample. Perhaps this problem should be investigated further, but its presence does not affect the test of significance unduly.

(iv) The residuals are independent of each other. In the case where there are separate single measurements on individuals, then there is no problem with independence. There is no reason to suppose that measurements made on one individual are likely to affect a different individual. There are two situations in which the assumption might be violated.

(1) If the observations are ordered in time.

Example from the literature

Figure 7.8(a) shows the monthly number of AIDS cases in the UK from January 1983 to December 1986, with the best-fit straight line.

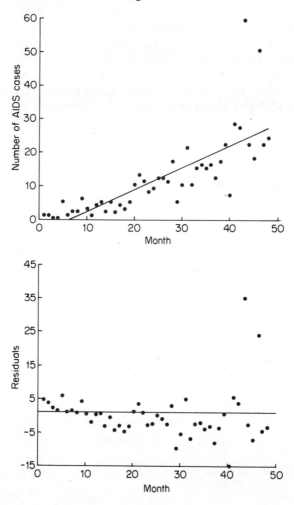

Figure 7.8   (a) A scatter plot of monthly number of AIDS cases in the UK from January 1983 to December 1986 against time, and (b) the residuals from linear regression against time

Figure 7.8(b) is a plot of the residuals from the best-fit line against time. It is clear from the figure that one positive residual is likely to be followed by another positive one and a negative residual is likely to be followed by another negative one. This suggests that the residuals are not random and so the model does not describe the data well and the tests of significance are not valid.

(2) If different numbers of observations are made on some individuals, but all observations are treated equally.

Example from the literature

Figure 7.9 shows the relationship between the percentage white-matter water content and longitudinal relaxation time, T_1, from a study by Bell *et al.* (1987).

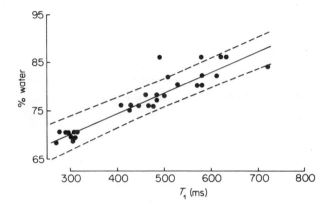

Figure 7.9   Percentage of water in the cortex and longitudinal relaxation time T_1 (after Bell *et al.*, 1987, with permission)

The authors refer to 19 patients in the study, and yet there are 30 points on the graph, so some of the patients must have had at least two observations. The regression equation is not estimated correctly in these circumstances, if all 30 observation pairs are included in the calculations of a and b in the manner described in Appendix A12.

A moment's thought should help persuade the reader. Suppose one conducted a survey of haemoglobin and age, making one observation per individual. Suppose there was one elderly woman with a high haemoglobin level, but the rest of the data showed little relationship between haemoglobin and age. On the spurious grounds that this relationship is 'interesting', a clinician could recall this woman 5 times for blood tests, to produce 5 extra points in the top right-hand section of the graph, and thus generate a statistically significant relationship.

The usual procedure to adopt for multiple measurements is to take an average for each individual and treat the averages as single observations.

(d) Do the assumptions matter?

The art in statistics occurs when deciding how far the assumptions can be stretched without providing a seriously misleading summary and when the procedure should be abandoned altogether and other methods tried. In general, lack of Normality of the residuals is unlikely to affect seriously the estimates of a regression equation, although Bland (1987) has pointed out that it may affect the standard errors and the size of the p-value. Similarly, a lack of constant variance of the residuals is unlikely to seriously affect the estimates, but again will have some influence on the final p-value.

In either case the advice would be to proceed, but with caution, particularly if the p-value is close to some critical value such as 0.05.

The lack of linearity is more serious, and would suggest either a transformation of the data before fitting the regression equation, or a model involving quadratic (squared) or higher terms using multiple regression (see Section 7.5).

Lack of independence of the residuals can also be serious. If the data form a time sequence, or if the data involve replications over individuals, a correct analysis may be difficult and expert advice should be sought.

(e) Regression and prediction

One of the major advantages of a regression equation over a correlation coefficient is that it enables one to predict values of the dependent variable.

Example from the literature

Campbell (1985) showed that one was able to predict the finishing time of an athlete running a half marathon from his resting pulse rate (RPR). Thus he showed that

$$\text{Finishing time} = 92 + 0.35 \times (\text{RPR} - 59).$$

That is, for every beat/minute above 59 beats/minute, the finishing time in the half marathon increased by 0.35 minutes.

In these situations it is important to be aware that the prediction equation is only valid within the range of the independent variable from which it was derived. Thus, in Campbell (1985) the range of resting pulse rates in the sample was 40 beats/min to 94 beats/min. It would be unwise to use the derived equation to predict a running speed of a runner where resting pulse was 110 beats/min.

There is no evidence that the linear relationship, which was true between 50 and 80 beats/min, will remain up until 100 beats/min. Confidence intervals for predictions obtained by linear regression are discussed by Altman and Gardner (1988).

7.4 COMPARISON OF ASSUMPTIONS BETWEEN CORRELATION AND REGRESSION

The tests of significance for a correlation coefficient and a regression coefficient yield identical t-statistics and p-values for a particular data set.

It is one of the nice coincidences in statistics that two completely different sets of assumptions lead to the same test of significance. This would seem logical since one would not expect to have a significant correlation in the absence of a significant regression effect. Unfortunately this has often led to a confusion between correlation and regression. However, the assumptions underlying the tests are quite different. The major difference is that in regression there is no stipulation about the distribution of the independent variable x. It is often the case that the x's are determined by the experimenter. In the anaemia survey of Campbell et al. (1985) one might choose fixed numbers of women in specified age groups; in a laboratory survey one might be interested in the responses of patients to fixed levels of a drug chosen by the experimenter. However, choosing fixed values for the x's violates the assumption underlying the correlation coefficient, namely that the x's have a Normal distribution.

Example

Selecting only the 6 women with a PCV of 35% and less, and the 3 women with 50% and more, in Table 7.1, the correlation coefficient between haemoglobin and PCV becomes $r = 0.78$ as compared to 0.67 for the full data set.

In regression it is perfectly valid to have x variables that can take only the values 0 and 1. These are clearly very far from being Normally distributed.

For a given data set one can always calculate both the correlation coefficient and the regression line. However, as has been seen, one will usually wish to quote only one or the other. The following are guidelines to help the reader decide which.

(i) Can one of the variables be predetermined, or altered? In that case quote regression coefficients.
(ii) Does one wish to summarise the strength of an association? If so, quote the correlation coefficient.
(iii) Is it clear which variable is the dependent one? If it is clear, then one would quote the regression coefficients, unless one also wanted a measure of the strength of the relationship. However, if the independent variable is clearly not Normally distributed it is necessary to use regression.

7.5 MULTIPLE REGRESSION

(a) The multiple regression equation

Life is rarely simple, and outcome variables in medical research are usually affected by a multitude of factors. Fortunately the simple linear regression situation with one independent variable is easily extended to multiple regression. In that case the corresponding model is

$$y_i = \alpha + \beta_1 x_{1i} + \beta_2 x_{2i} + \ldots + \beta_k x_{ki}$$

where x_{1i} is the first independent variable, x_{2i} is the second, and so on up to the kth independent variable x_{ki}.

The term α is the intercept or constant term. It is the value of y_i when all the independent variables are zero. The regression coefficients $\beta_1, \ldots \beta_k$ are again estimated by minimising the sum of the squares of the differences from the observed and predicted outcome variables, y_i and Y_i. Although the variables $x_{1i}, \ldots, x_{ki}$ are termed the independent variables, it should be noted that this is a misnomer, since they need not be independent of one another. Although it is not essential that clinicians understand the computational details of multiple regression, it is such a commonly used technique that they will need to be able to understand both computer output from a multiple regression calculation and read papers which use the results of multiple regression.

(b) Uses of multiple regression

(i) To look for relationships between continuous variables, allowing for a third variable. In the examples above we found a significant correlation between haemoglobin level and PCV, and a significant regression between haemoglobin level and age. This stimulates us to ask: Is the relationship between haemoglobin and PCV only apparent because they both increase with age? In other words, does age act as a *confounding variable*?

Example

The output from a multiple regression program of two independent variables age and PCV on haemoglobin is given in Table 7.2.

Table 7.2   Output from multiple regression, Hb against age and PCV

Dependent variable: Haemoglobin level

Variable		Regression coefficient	SE	t-value	p-value
Constant	a	5.24	1.21	4.34	0.004
Age	b_1	0.110	0.016	6.74	0.0001
PCV	b_2	0.097	0.033	2.98	0.0085

In Table 7.2 the constant 5.24 is the estimated value of the α intercept of the equation. It is the haemoglobin level estimated for someone with age and PCV of zero and, as is often the case, has little real interpretation since patients of age and PCV values of zero are rare. However, it is usually produced by multiple regression programs and is needed in the prediction equation. Age and PCV are the two independent variables and the regression coefficients are the estimates of the βs in the regression equation. We therefore write

$$\text{Predicted haemoglobin} = 5.24 + 0.110 \, (\text{Age}) + 0.097 \, (\text{PCV})$$

The interpretation of the regression coefficient associated with PCV is that for a given age, haemoglobin increases by 0.097 g/dl for every unit increase in PCV. This is in contrast to our earlier calculations in which $b = 0.121$ but age was not taken into account in the relation.

Every parameter estimate has associated with it a standard error (SE). The corresponding t-value is the regression coefficient estimate divided by its SE and the degrees of freedom are given by the number of observations minus the number of estimated parameters. In this case, df$= 20 - 3 = 17$. From these we can derive the p-value by use of Table T2. These are given in Table 7.2. The p-values correspond to the probability of observing that particular regression coefficient, or one more extreme, on the null hypothesis assumption that the true regression coefficient is in fact zero.

Since the coefficient associated with PCV is still highly significant, the conclusion is that haemoglobin and PCV are related even when age is taken into account.

(ii) To adjust for differences in confounding factors between groups.

Example

Suppose an investigator wished to test whether, on average, women of Table 7.1 who have experienced the menopause, have a different haemoglobin level than women who have not. The mean and standard deviation of haemoglobin for pre-menopausal women are 12.29 and 1.57 g/dl, whereas those for post-menopausal women are 16.36 and 0.63 respectively.

A simple *t*-test as described in Chapter 6 yields a difference between the pre- and post-menopausal women of -4.07 g/dl ($t = -7.3$, df= 18, $p < 0.001$), which is very highly significant. However, clearly women who have experienced the menopause will be older than women who have not. If there were a steady rise in haemoglobin with age, this might account for the difference observed and not the menopausal status itself.

Example

Menopausal status can be added to a multiple regression equation which includes age by means of a *dummy variable*. Such a variable takes the value 1 if the woman is post-menopausal and 0 if she is not. The output from the multiple regression program is given in Table 7.3.

Table 7.3   Output from multiple regression Hb against age and menopausal status

Dependent variable: Haemoglobin level

Variable		Regression coefficient	SE	*t*-value	*p*-value
Constant	a	11.62	1.99	5.81	<0.001
Age	b_1	0.081	0.033	2.41	0.03
Menopause	b_2	1.88	1.03	1.82	0.08

Note that the size of the coefficient associated with age has reduced from that of Table 7.2. This is because menopausal status is associated with age and age and menopausal status are being fitted simultaneously. The interpretation of the coefficient associated with the variable menopause is that, allowing for age, women who are post-menopausal have a haemoglobin level 1.88 g/dl higher than women who are not. However, the corresponding 95% confidence interval for β_2 with 17 df is

$$1.88 \ - \ t_{0.05} \ \times \ 1.03 \quad \text{to} \quad 1.88 \ + \ t_{0.05} \ \times \ 1.03$$

or -0.28 to 4.04. This interval includes zero, and so the conclusion made previously that there was a difference between pre- and post-menopausal women is largely discounted. It is the relative ages of the women in the two groups that accounts for the difference in haemoglobin levels.

This analysis assumes that the relationship between haemoglobin and age remains the same in women before and after the menopause. This assumption could be tested, but more complicated analyses are required.

Note that these are not the best data to answer the question: 'Do post-menopausal women have a higher haemoglobin level than pre-menopausal women?' For a cross-sectional study it would be better to collect data from women who are immediately pre- or post-menopausal. Better still would be a longitudinal study which measured haemoglobin levels in women before and after their menopause.

7.6 POINTS WHEN READING THE LITERATURE

(1) When a correlation coefficient is calculated, is the relationship likely to be linear?
(2) Are the variables likely to be Normally distributed?
(3) Is a plot of the data in the paper?
(4) If a significant correlation is obtained and the causation inferred, could there be a third factor, not measured, which is jointly correlated with the other two, and so account for their association?
(5) Remember correlation does not necessarily imply causation.
(6) If a scatter plot is given to support a linear regression, is the variability of the points about the line roughly the same over the range of the independent variable? If not, then perhaps some transformation of the variables is necessary before computing the regression line.
(7) If predictions are given, are they made from within the range of the observed values of the independent variable?

Chapter 8

The randomised controlled trial

Summary

This chapter emphasises the importance of the randomised clinical trials in evaluating alternative treatments. The importance of having a study protocol and the necessary requisites for estimating the appropriate size of a trial are described. Checklists of points to consider when designing, analysing and reading the reports describing a clinical trial are included.

8.1 INTRODUCTION

The human body is a very complex organism whose functioning is far from being completely understood. It is often difficult or impossible to predict from previous knowledge the exact reaction that a diseased individual will have to a new therapy. Although medical science might suggest that a new treatment is efficacious, it is only when it is tried in practice that any realistic assessment of its efficacy and the presence of any adverse side-effects can be obtained. No two individuals are alike, and it is only on rare occasions that a new therapy can cure every patient who has the particular disease. In general some patients will benefit from therapy and some will not.

Thus it is necessary to do comparative studies to compare the new treatment against the standard treatment. It should be emphasised, however, that randomised controlled trials are relevant to other areas of medical research; for example, in the evaluation of screening procedures, alternative formats for health education and contraceptive efficacy.

Although this book is about the use of statistics in all branches of medical activity, this chapter is devoted to the randomised clinical trial because it has a central role in the development of new therapies. The topic of clinical trials is described in extensive detail in specialist books by Pocock (1983) and Schwartz, Flamant and Lellouch (1980).

Some points concerning the design of clinical trials have been made in Chapter 2 and here a two-group parallel design, similar to that shown in Figure 2.1 is used for illustration.

8.2 DESIGN FEATURES

(a) The need for a control group

Chapter 2 discussed the hazards of 'before-and-after' type studies, in which physicians simply stop using the standard treatment and start using the new. In any situation in which a new therapy is under investigation, one important question is whether it is any better than the currently best available for the particular condition. If the new therapy is indeed better then, all other considerations being equal, it would seem reasonable to give all future patients with the condition the new therapy. But how well are the patients doing with the current therapy? Once a therapy is in routine use it is not generally monitored to the same rigorous standards as it was during its development. So although the current best therapy may have been carefully tested many years prior to the proposed new study, changes in medical practice may have ensued in the interim. It could well be that some of these changes have influenced patient outcome. The possibility of such changes makes it imperative that the new therapy is tested alongside the old. In addition, although there may be a presumption of improved efficacy, the new therapy may turn out to be not as good as the old. It therefore becomes very important to redetermine the efficacy of the standard treatment under current conditions.

(b) Treatment choice and follow-up

When designing a clinical trial one must have firm objectives in view. Thus clearly different and well-defined alternative treatment regimens are required. The criteria for patient entry should be clear and measures of efficacy should be prespecified and unambiguously determined for each patient. All patients entered into a trial and randomised to treatment should be followed up in the same manner, irrespective of whether or not the treatment is continuing for that individual patient. Thus a patient who refuses a second injection in a drug study should be monitored as closely as one who agreed to the injection. From considerations of sample size (see Section 8.4) it is usually preferable to compare at most two treatments, although, clearly, there are situations in which more than two can be evaluated efficiently. One such study is that of McMaster, Nichols and Machin (1985) referred to in Chapter 2, which describes the comparison of four forms of breast self-examination teaching material.

(c) The need for random assignment of treatments to patients

Subjects should be allocated at random to the alternative available treatments. The study protocol will clearly define the patient entry criteria for a particular trial. After the physician has determined that the patient is indeed eligible for the study, there is one extra question to answer. This is: 'Are each of the treatments under study appropriate for this particular patient?' If the answer is 'Yes', the patient is then randomised. If 'No', the patient is not included in the study and would receive treatment according to the discretion of the physician. It is therefore important that the physician does not know, at this stage, which of the treatments the patient is going to receive if included in the study. The randomisation list should therefore be prepared and held by separate members of the study team or distributed to the clinician in charge in sealed envelopes to be opened only once the patient is confirmed as eligible for the trial.

(d) Blind assessment

Just as the physician who determines eligibility to the study should be blind to the actual treatment that the patient would receive, any assessment of the patient should preferably be 'blind'! Thus one should separate the assessment process from the treatment process if this is at all possible. To obtain an even more objective view of efficacy it is desirable to have the patient 'blind' to which of the treatments he or she is receiving. Clinical trials are concerned with real and not abstract situations so it is recognised that the ideal 'double-blind' situation may not be possible or even desirable in all circumstances. If there is a choice. however, the maximum degree of 'blindness' should be adhered to. A 'double-blind' study requires careful monitoring since treatment-related adverse side-effects are a possibility in any trial and the attendant physician may need to be able to have immediate access to the actual treatment given should an emergency arise.

(e) 'Pragmatic' versus 'explanatory' trials

Schwartz, Flamant and Lellouch (1980) draw a useful distinction between trials that aim to determine the exact pharmacological action of a drug ('explanatory' trials) and trials that aim to determine the efficacy of a drug as used in day-to-day clinical practice ('pragmatic' trials). There are many factors besides lack of efficacy that can interfere with the action of a drug; for example, if a drug is unpalatable, patients may not like its taste and therefore not take it. Explanatory trials often require some measure of patient compliance, perhaps by means of blood samples, to determine whether the drug was actually taken by the patient. Such trials need to be conducted in tightly controlled situations. Patients found not to have complied with the prescribed dose schedule may be excluded from analysis. On the other hand, pragmatic trials lead to analysis by 'intention to treat'. Thus once patients are randomised to receive a particular treatment they are analysed as if they have received it, whether or not they did so in practice. This will reflect the likely action of the drug in clinical practice, where even when a drug is prescribed there is no guarantee that the patient will take it.

8.3 THE PROTOCOL

The protocol is a formal document specifying how the trial is to be conducted. It will usually be necessary to write a protocol if the investigator is going to submit the trial to a grant-giving body for support and/or to an ethical committee for approval. However, there are also good practical reasons why one should prepare one in any case. The protocol provides the reference document for clinicians entering patients into clinical trials. The main content requirements of a study protocol are as follows:

(1) *Introduction, background and general aims*. This would describe the justification for the trial and, for example, the expected pharmacological action of the drug under test and its possible side-effects.

(2) *Specific objectives*. This should describe the main hypothesis or hypotheses being tested. For example, the new drug may be required to acheive the same survival experience as the standard yet have fewer unwanted side-effects.

(3) *Patient selection*. Suitable patients need to be clearly identified. It is important to stress that all treatments under test must be appropriate for the patients recruited.

(4) *Personnel and roles*. The personnel who have overall responsibility for the trial and who have the day-to-day responsibility for the patient management have to be identified. The respective roles of physician, surgeon, radiotherapist, oncologist and pathologist may have to be clarified and organised in a trial concerned with a new treatment for cancer. The individual responsible for the coordination of the data will need to be specified.

(5) *Adverse events*. Clear note should be made of who to contact in the case of a clinical emergency and arrangements made for the monitoring of adverse events.

(6) *Trial design and randomisation*. A brief description of the essential features of the design of the trial should be included preferably with a diagram (see Figure 2.1 for one example). It is useful also to include an indication of the time of visits for treatment, assessment and follow-up of the patients. There should also be a clear statement of how randomisation is carried out.

(7) *Trial observations and assessments*. Details of the necessary observations and their timing need to be provided. The main outcome variables should be identified so that the clinician involved can ensure that these are assessed in each patient.

(8) *Treatment schedules*. Clear and unambiguous descriptions of the actual treatment schedules should be given. These could be very simple instructions in the case of prescribing a new antibiotic for otitis media or be very complex in a chemotherapy regimen for osteosarcoma.

(9) *Trial supplies*. It is clearly important that there are sufficient supplies of the new drug available and that those responsible for the dispensing the drug and other supplies are identified.

(10) *Patient consent*. The method of obtaining patient consent should be summarised and, if appropriate, a suggested consent form included.

(11) *Required size of study*. The anticipated treatment effect, the test size and power (see Section 6.9) should be specified and the number of patients that need to be recruited estimated. It is often useful to include an estimate of the patient accrual rate.

(12) *Forms and data handling*. Details of how the data are to be recorded should be provided. It is usual for a copy of the data forms to be attached to the protocol.

(13) *Statistical analysis*. This would give a brief description of how the data are to be analysed. It would include the tests which are to be used and whether one- or two-sided comparisons are to be utilised.

(14) *Protocol deviations*. Treatment details are required for patients who deviate from or refuse the protocol therapy. Clearly a particular therapy may be refused by a patient during the course of the trial so alternative treatment schedules may be suggested. This section may also describe dose modifications permitted within the protocol which are dependent on patient response or the appearance of some side effect.

8.4 STUDY SIZE

The appropriate number of patients to be recruited to a study is dependent on four components, each of which requires careful consideration by the investigating team.

(a) Control group response

It is first necessary to estimate the response of patients to the control or standard therapy. This will be denoted by π_1. Experience of other patients with the particular disease or the medical literature concerned may provide a reasonably precise estimate for this figure in many circumstances.

(b) The anticipated benefit

It is also necessary to postulate the size of the anticipated response in patients receiving the new treatment, denoted by π_2. Thus one might know that approximately 40% of patients are likely to respond to the control therapy, and if this could be improved to 50% by the new therapy then a clinically worthwhile benefit would have been demonstrated. Thus the anticipated benefit $\delta = \pi_2 - \pi_1 = 10\%$. Of course it is not yet known if the new therapy will have such benefit but the study should be planned so that if such an advantage does exist there will be a reasonable chance of detecting it.

It should be noted that the Greek letters have been used for the parameters in a different way than in earlier chapters. Here π_1 is the value we think that the response rate in the patients receiving the control treatment will be. We then conduct the clinical trial and obtain p_1 which is then taken as the estimate of π_1. Similarily π_2 is the anticipated response rate in patients who will receive the new therapy. Once the trial has been conducted we can calculate p_2 and we hope that it will be at least as large as π_2.

(c) Significance level

The third requirement is the two-sided significance level, usually denoted by α, to be used in formal tests of significance or confidence intervals. In many studies a p-value of less than 5% is taken as indicative of rejecting the null hypothesis that the two treatments are equally effective. Arguments have been given elsewhere in this book against the rigid use of significance tests. Thus we have discouraged the use of statements such as: 'the null hypothesis is rejected $p < 0.05$', or worse, 'we accept the null hypothesis $p > 0.05$'. However, in calculating sample size it is convenient to think in terms of a significance test and to specify the test size α in advance.

(d) Power

The last item of information required is the acceptable false negative or type II error rate that is judged to be reasonable. This is the probability of accepting the null hypothesis of no difference between treatments, when the anticipated benefit in fact exists. This is usually denoted by β. Experience of others suggests that in practice the type II error rate is often set at a maximum value of $\beta = 20\%$. More usually this is alternatively expressed as setting the power of the test as $1 - \beta = 80\%$.

For any combination of the four basic items there is a corresponding number of patients per group. Figure 8.1 shows how the number of patients per treatment group changes with respect to π_1 and δ for fixed $\alpha = 5\%$ and $\beta = 80\%$.

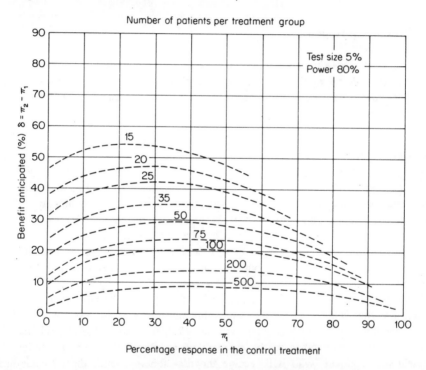

Figure 8.1   Change in sample size for the comparison of two proportions

Thus for $\pi_1 = 50\%$, the number of patients to be recruited to each treatment decreases from approximately 500, 100, 50 to 25 as δ increases from 10, 20, 30 to 40%. If α or β are decreased then the necessary number of subjects increases. The eventual study size depends on these arbitrarily chosen values in a critical way. There is no way to avoid them, however.

Example from the literature

In the study conducted by Familiari *et al.* (1981) (see Table 6.1), two drugs for the treatment of peptic ulcer were compared. The percentage of ulcers healed by pirenzepine and trithiozine were 76.7 and 58.1% respectively.

Suppose that the trial is to be conducted again but now with the benefit of hindsight. The response to trithiozine in the study was approximately 60% and that to pirenzepine approximately 75%. These provide the anticipated response rate for the control treatment as $\pi_1 = 60\%$ and an expected benefit, $\delta = \pi_2 - \pi_1 = 15\%$. Setting $\alpha = 5\%$ and $1 - \beta = 80\%$, then Figure 8.1 suggests approximately $m = 150$ patients per group. Thus a total of 300 patients would be required for the confirmatory study.

It is usual at the planning stage of a study to investigate differences that would arise if the assumptions used in the calculations were altered. In particular we may have overestimated the response rate of the controls. If π_1 is in fact closer to 50% than 60%, then, keeping $\delta = 15\%$, there is a change in our estimate of the required number of patients from 150 to approximately 170 per group. As a consequence we may have to be concerned about the reliability of this estimate. In situations where the outcome measure is continuous the number of patients required is not so sensitive to changes in the response rate of the control therapy.

In certain situations an investigator may only have access to a restricted number of patients for a particular trial. In this case the investigator reasonably ask: 'With an anticipated response rate π_1 in the controls, a difference in efficacy postulated to be δ, and assuming $\alpha = 5\%$, what is the power $1 - \beta$ of my proposed study?'. If the power is low, say 50%, the investigator may decide not to proceed further with the trial or may seek the help of other colleagues, perhaps in other centres, to recruit more patients to the trial and thereby increase the power to an acceptable value. This device of encouraging others to contribute to the collective attack on a clinically important question is used by, for example, the British Medical Research Council, the US National Institute of Health, and the World Health Organization.

Formulae for more precise calculations for the number of patients required to make comparisons of two proportions and for the comparison of two means are given in Appendix A15. Extensive examples and tables are given in the book by Machin and Campbell (1987) for these and other situations.

It is important to know that the number of patients per treatment group depends on the type of summary statistic being utilised. In general, studies in which data are continuous and can be summarised by a mean require fewer patients than those in which the response can only be assessed as either a success or failure. Survival time studies often require fewer events to be observed than those with purely binary endpoints.

8.5 ONE-SIDED COMPARISONS

In the peptic ulcer example, it may be that the investigator confidently anticipates that pirenzepine will achieve a higher response rate than trithiozine. If this is wrong and the opposite were in fact the case, there may be no further interest in this drug for therapy. Under such circumstances it may be argued in planning the trial that a one-sided alternative hypothesis is more appropriate. The only change in the equations to calculate the number of patients required is to replace α by 2α. In this example, keeping the other three components of the calculation unchanged, the required number of patients per group is reduced from 150 to 120. This would then give a total of 240 patients rather than 300 for the intended new study. In either event the patient numbers are much larger than the 61 recruited for the published study.

If a one-sided test is specified in the protocol but a result in the other direction is obtained, then even if it is tested and found to be formally 'statistically significant', it should not be taken as evidence of a real effect in that direction. This is because at the planning stage the investigators ruled out this possibility. The result is therefore so unexpected that it could well be explained as an occasion when a false positive is known to have occurred!

8.6 SURVIVAL COMPARISONS

The major outcome variable in some clinical trials is the time from randomisation to a specified critical event. Examples include patient survival time, the time a kidney graft remains patent, length of time that an indwelling cannula remains *in situ* or the time in remission from a recurrent disease. In such situations the efficacy of treatments being compared in a randomised clinical trial might be summarised by the median survival times of the patients in the various treatment groups.

Even when the final outcome is not survival time from randomisation to death, the techniques employed with such data are conveniently termed *survival analysis* methods. The length of time from entry to the study to when the critical event occurs is called the *survival time*.

Although survival time is a continuous variable one cannot use a standard *t*-test for analysis as described in Chapter 6. There are two reasons for this:

(i) The distribution of survival times is unlikely to be Normal and it may not be possible to find a transformation that will make it so.

(ii) The presence of *censored* observations.

Censored observations arise in patients for whom the critical event has not yet occurred. Thus although some of the patients recruited to a particular trial may have died and their survival time is calculable, others may still be alive or lost to follow-up. The time from randomisation to the last date the live patient was examined is known as the censored survival time, as has been described in Chapter 4. Censored observations can arise in three ways: (a) the patient is known to be still alive when the trial analysis is carried out; (b) the patient was known to be alive at some past follow-up, but the investigator has since lost trace of him; or (c) the patient has died of some cause totally unrelated to the disease in question.

One method of analysis of survival data is to specify in advance a fixed time period at which comparisons are to be made and then compare proportions of patients whose survival times exceed this time period. For example, one may compare the proportion of patients alive at one year in the two treatment groups. This ignores the individual survival times and can be very wasteful of the available information.

However, techniques have been developed to deal with survival data which can take account of the information provided by censored observations. Such data can be displayed using a *Kaplan–Meier* survival plot, as shown, for example in Figure 4.9 and group comparisons can be made using the *logrank* test. These techniques are described in Appendix A17.

Example from the literature

Chant, Turner and Machin (1984) compared two drugs metronidazole and ampicillin, which are used to avoid post-operative wound infection, using a randomised trial in adult patients undergoing appendicectomy. One of the major outcome variables was the length of the post-operative fever actually experienced by the patients.

There were no censored observations in their study and they summarised their findings by use of the geometric mean number of days of fever in each group.

Example from the literature

Sutton *et al.* (1987) compared time from diagnosis to recurrence of breast cancer in women with early disease and with either negative, low or high progesterone receptor status.

The corresponding Kaplan–Meier survival curves are shown in Figure 8.2. The results revealed that progesterone receptor status was a significant predictor of recurrence.

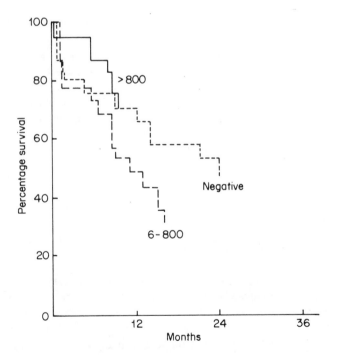

Figure 8.2 Kaplan–Meier survival curves for time to disease recurrence by receptor status in 65 patients with early breast cancer, with either negative, low or high progesterone receptor from the time of first local or distant recurrence. There were 24, 23 and 18 patients in each respective progesterone receptor group, $p < 0.05$, logrank test (after Sutton *et al.*, 1987)

8.7 INTERIM ANALYSIS AND SEQUENTIAL TRIALS

In many trials patients are not all available at the start of the study but are recruited steadily through time. Thus the outcome of the earlier patients may be known before the later patients have been recruited. In such cases it is tempting for an investigator to analyse the data obtained to date. Indeed one could argue that ethically one should do so in the best interests of patients as it may turn out that there is sufficient evidence to conclude that the new treatment is markedly better than the standard, in which case it would no longer be ethical to use the old treatment on patients about to be recruited.

The statistical problem is that continual looks at the data result in too many tests on much the same data. This has the effect of increasing the chance that a type I error is made. Thus one is more likely to conclude there is an effect even when it is in fact absent. The compromise solution is usually to allow what are known as *interim analyses* at intervals prespecified in the protocol as the data accumulates. At each interim analysis a much lower significance level than the α specified in the protocol is used. For example, one might specify that five interim analyses are to be performed during the course of the trial, in which one would only declare a result significant if the p-value is less than $0.05/5 = 0.01$. The implication of a significant result is that once declared, recruitment to the study ceases. If no interim analysis is declared significant, patients continue to be recruited until the target recruitment is obtained. The eventual analysis of all the data is then done with a test size of α. Pocock (1983) gives tables showing different methods of allocating significance levels for various design and numbers of interim analyses.

An extreme situation occurs when the treatment outcome of a patient is known very quickly. Thus one might wish to monitor the trial as each individual result is known. An example might be a randomised trial of two anaesthetics where the outcome is the level of nausea experienced in the immediate post-operative period by the patients. Such trials can be analysed using a technique termed *sequential analysis*. It can be shown that a sequential design can reduce the number of patients required in a trial, but there are problems with providing valid estimates of the effects and confidence intervals. It is worth consulting a statistician if a sequential trial is contemplated. The general methodology is quite technical and is described by Whitehead (1983).

8.8 ETHICAL CONSIDERATIONS

In planning a study involving patients, it is not sensible to embark on the study if the chance of detecting the anticipated difference is small. The medical literature contains the results of many small studies which are declared as 'not significant' and so mistakenly implying that the two treatments are in fact equivalent. This is often the consequence of conducting a study of inadequate size. Gore and Altman (1982) have argued that such studies are unethical. They may, for example, bring discomfort to a patient yet not be large enough to convincingly demonstrate the advantages of a new therapy. This is not to say that all trials must be large, and small trials can provide 'ball-park' estimates of the effects of treatment and rule out grandiose claims. A discussion of these points is given by Powell-Tuck *et al.* (1986).

8.9 CHECKLISTS FOR THE DESIGN AND ANALYSIS OF TRIALS

A guide to the useful points to look for when considering a new trial are given by checklists such as those of Gardner, Machin and Campbell (1986). Although these lists were primarily developed for assessing the quality of manuscripts submitted for publication, they clearly cover aspects worthy of consideration at the planning stage of a trial. The main features of their checklists include:

(a) Design

(1) Are the objectives clearly formulated?
(2) Are the diagnostic criteria for entry to the trial clear?
(3) Are there sufficient potential patients?
(4) Are the treatments (or interventions) well defined?
(5) Are the method and reason for randomisation well understood?
(6) Is the treatment planned to commence immediately following randomisation?
(7) Is the maximum degree of blindness being used?
(8) Are the outcome measures appropriate?
(9) Are the outcome measures clearly defined?
(10) How has the study size been justified?
(11) What arrangements have been made for collecting, recording and analysis of the data?
(12) Has appropriate follow-up of the patients been organised?
(13) Are important prognostic variables recorded?
(14) Are side-effects of treatment anticipated?
(15) Are many patient drop-outs anticipated?

(b) Analysis and presentation

(1) Are the statistical procedures used adequately described or referenced?
(2) Are the statistical procedures appropriate?
(3) Have the potential prognostic variables been adequately considered?
(4) Is the statistical presentation satisfactory?
(5) Are any graphs clear and appropriately labelled?
(6) Are confidence intervals given for the main results?
(7) Are the conclusions drawn from the statistical analysis justified?

8.10 POINTS WHEN READING THE LITERATURE

(1) Go through the checklists described above
(2) Check whether the trial is indeed truly randomised. Alternate patient allocation to treatments is not randomised allocation.

(3) Check the diagnostic criteria for entry. Many treatments are tested in a restricted group of patients even though they could then be prescribed for another. For example, one exclusion criterion for trials of non-steroidal anti-inflammatory drugs (NSAIDs) is often extreme age, yet the drugs once evaluated are often prescribed for elderly patients.

(4) Is the actual size of the treatment effect reported?

(5) Does the Abstract correctly report what was found in the paper?

Chapter 9

Designed observational studies

Summary

The incidence rate and the prevalence are statistics used to describe disease in a population. The two main types of study are cohort studies and case-control studies. The main summary statistics used in a cohort study are the relative risk and the attributable risk. In a case-control study the main summary statistic is the odds ratio. In many situations the odds ratio can be shown to give a good approximation to the relative risk. The standardised mortality ratio is a statistic used to compare mortality in groups whose age distributions may be different.

9.1 INTRODUCTION

In Chapter 8 and earlier, it was emphasised that the essential feature of a clinical trial was the random allocation of treatment to subjects. However, in many situations where an investigator is looking for an association between exposure to a risk factor and subsequent disease, it is not possible to randomly allocate exposure to subjects; you cannot insist that some people smoke and others do not, or randomly expose some industrial workers to radiation. Thus studies relating exposure to outcome are often observational; the investigator simply observes what happens and does not intervene. The options under the control of the investigator are restricted to the choice of subjects, whether to follow them retrospectively or prospectively, and the size of the sample. If the observations are continuous, then the techniques of regression described in Chapter 7 are used to investigate associations. Very often, however, the observations are discrete, or can be made so. For example a population may be exposed to varying levels of radiation but it is often useful to group them into just two categories such as 'slight exposure' and 'severe exposure'. Similarly, although subjects may vary in the severity of disease that develops it is often convenient to simply classify them into either those that have or those that do not have a disease. In such a situation the techniques described in this chapter are relevant. As in regression, the major problem in the interpretation of observational studies is that although an association between exposure and disease can be observed, this does not necessarily imply a causal relationship. For example, many studies have shown that smoking is associated with subsequent lung cancer. It has been argued, however, that some people are genetically susceptible to lung cancer, and this same gene predisposes them to smoke! Factors that are related to both the exposure to a risk factor and the subsequent outcome are called *confounding* factors. In observational studies it is always possible to think of potential confounding factors that might explain away an argument for causality. However, some methods for strengthening the causality argument are given later in the chapter.

9.2 RATES

A *rate* is defined as the number of events, for example deaths or cases of disease, per unit of population, in a particular time span. To calculate a rate the following are needed:

(1) A defined period of time (for example, a calendar year).
(2) A defined population, with an accurate estimate of the size of the population during the defined period.
(3) The number of events occurring over the period.

One example of a rate is the *crude mortality rate* (CMR) for a particular year, which is given by

$$\text{CMR} = \frac{\text{Number of deaths occurring in year}}{\text{Mid-year population}} \times 1000$$

It is important to remember that rates must refer to a specific period of time. They are usually referred to as events per 1000 or 100000 since it is much easier to think of 12 deaths per 1000 than 0.012 deaths per individual.

If a particular age group is specified, the *age-specific mortality rate* (ASMR) is obtained as

$$\text{ASMR} = \frac{\text{Number of deaths occurring in specified age group}}{\text{Mid-year number in that age group}} \times 1000$$

The *incidence* rate refers to the number of new cases of a particular disease that develop during a specified time interval. The *prevalence* (which is strictly not a rate since no time period is specified) refers to the number of cases of a disease that exist at a specified point in time.

9.3 COHORT STUDY

(a) Notation

The design of cohort studies is discussed in Chapter 2 and the progress of a cohort study is described in Figure 2.3. Table 9.1 gives the notation for the statistics used to describe a cohort study in this chapter.

Table 9.1   Notation for a cohort study

	Number of subjects who develop disease in follow-up	Number of subjects who do not develop disease in follow-up	Total
Exposed to risk factor	a	b	$a + b$
Not exposed to risk factor	c	d	$c + d$

Example from the literature

Piedras *et al.* (1983) describe a one-year follow-up of 30 women, after the insertion of an intrauterine device. They were looking for factors that might predict which women might become anaemic. Serum ferritin and haemoglobin were measured at the start of the survey, and after one year. Women were divided by whether their serum ferritin was above or below 20 μg/l, anaemia defined as a haemoglobin level below 13.8 g/dl, The results, summarised in Table 9.2, show number of women who develop anaemia by level of serum ferritin.

Table 9.2   Numbers of women in cohort study of serum ferritin and anaemia

	Anaemic at 2nd survey	Not anaemic at 2nd survey	Total
Serum ferritin $< 20\,\mu$g/l 1st survey	7	8	15
Serum ferritin $\geq 20\,\mu$g/l 1st survey	2	13	15

Source: Piedras *et al.* (1983).

In this study the risk factor is having a serum ferritin level below 20 μg/l and the disease is anaemia.

(b) The relative risk

The *risk* of an event is the probability that an event will occur within a stated period of time. Thus from Table 9.1, the risk of developing the disease within the follow-up time is $a/(a + b)$ for the exposed population and $c/(c + d)$ for the unexposed population. In the example from Piedras *et al.*, the risk of becoming anaemic in one year is 7/15 for the low-ferritin group and 2/15 for the high-ferritin group. The *relative risk* (RR) is the ratio of these two, that is

$$RR = a(c + d)/\{c(a + b)\}$$

From Table 9.2, we get that the relative risk is 3.5. This is interpreted as meaning that a woman is more than 3 times more likely to become anaemic if her serum ferritin is below 20 μg/l at the commencement of IUD use.

(c) The population attributable risk

If smoking increases the risk of anaemia by 4 and low ferritin by 3.5, it is not necessarily correct to infer that smoking is responsible for more anaemic women than is low serum ferritin. If very few women smoked, the effect of smoking on the health of the population is not going to be large, however serious the consequences to the individual. The effect of a risk factor on community health is related to both relative risk and the percentage of the population exposed to the risk factor and this can be measured by the *attributable risk* (AR).

The terminology is not standard, but following Armitage and Berry (1987) let I_P be the incidence of a disease in the population and I_E and I_{NE} be the incidence in the exposed and not exposed respectively. Then the excess incidence attributable to the risk factor is simply $I_P - I_{NE}$ and the *population attributable risk* is

$$AR = (I_P - I_{NE})/I_P$$

that is, the percentage of the population risk that can be associated with the risk factor. Some authors define the excess risk as $I_E - I_{NE}$ and the population attributable risk as $(I_E - I_{NE})/I_{NE}$, but the first definition has the advantage of greater logical consistency.

If we define $\theta_E = (a + b)/N$ to be the proportion of the population of size N exposed to the risk factor then, it can be shown that

$$AR = \frac{\theta_E(RR - 1)}{1 + \theta_E(RR - 1)}$$

The advantage of this formula is that it enables the attributable risk to be calculated directly from the relative risk, and the proportion of the population exposed to the risk factor. Both of these can be estimated from cohort studies and also from case-control studies in certain circumstances when the controls are a random sample of the population. Thus, in the example above, $\theta_E = 15/30 = 0.5$, relative risk RR = 3.5 and so AR= 0.5 $\times$ 2.5/(1 + 0.5 $\times$ 2.5) = 0.55. That is, 55% of women have anaemia as a consequence of having a low serum ferritin when the IUD is fitted. Since the low and high ferritin groups are of equal size $((a + b) = (c + d))$ this result can be easily verified from the fact that the excess of anaemia cases in the low serum ferritin group is $7 - 2 = 5$, and as a proportion of all cases this is $5/9 = 55\%$.

(d) Why quote a relative risk?

The relative risk provides a convenient summary of the outcome of a cohort study. It is independent of the prevalence of the disease and so is more stable than the individual risks. For example, if the intrauterine device was used on a different population of women, the incidence of anaemia may be different. However, the incidence of anaemia is likely to be equally affected in the high and low serum ferritin groups, and so the relative risk of anaemia with a low serum ferritin remains unaltered. Also, it is often the case that if a factor in addition to the principal one under study acts independently on the disease process, the joint relative risk is just the product of the two relative risks. Thus if smokers, after the insertion of an intrauterine device, had a relative risk of 4 of developing anaemia compared with non-smokers, then the risk of anaemia among smokers with low serum ferritin is likely to be $4 \times 3.5 = 14$. If smoking data were available to the investigators, clearly this result could be verified.

Example from the literature

The Royal College of General Practitioners (1981) reported on a cohort study of women who used oral contraceptives. They report that the relative risk of death from circulatory disease for a woman who smokes is 2.0. The relative risk of death from circulatory disease for a non-smoker who takes oral contraceptives is 3.2 . If the two effects are multiplicative we would expect relative risk for a woman who smokes and takes oral contraceptives to be $2.0 \times 3.2 = 6.4$. In fact for a woman who smokes and takes oral contraceptives the observed relative risk is 5.1, which is not quite what one would expect if the two effects acted multiplicatively on the relative risks.

9.4 CASE-CONTROL STUDY

(a) Unmatched study

The design of case-control studies is discussed in Chapter 2. Table 9.3 gives the notation for the statistics used to describe unmatched case-control studies.

Table 9.3 Notation for an unmatched case-control study

	Cases (with disease)	Controls (without disease)
Exposed	a	b
Not exposed	c	d
Total	$a + c$	$b + d$

Example from the literature

Vessey *et al.* (1983) describe a case-control study of oral contraceptives and breast cancer. The cases were of recently diagnosed and histologically proven breast cancer in women aged 16–50 years, in certain hospitals. The controls were married women inpatients in the same hospital, who had certain acute medical or surgical conditions. The control women were interviewed in exactly the same way as the cases. The interview was conducted by a nurse or trained social worker and obtained social, medical, obstetric and contraceptive histories. The results of the study are summarised in Table 9.4.

Table 9.4   Results of unmatched case-control study of oral contraceptives and breast cancer

Oral Contraceptives	Cases	Controls
Ever Used	537	554
Never Used	639	622
Total	1176	1176

Source: Vessey *et al.* (1983).

We are interested in the relative risk of breast cancer in women taking oral contraceptives, but cannot get it directly in a case-control study. Instead we calculate what is known as the odds ratio for exposure and disease. The *odds* of an event is the ratio of the probability of occurrence of an event to the probability of non-occurrence. The *odds ratio* (OR) is the ratio of two odds. From Table 9.3, given that a subject has a disease, the odds of having been exposed are a/c; given that a subject does not have a disease, the odds of having been exposed are b/d. Then the odds ratio is OR= ad/bc.

An odds ratio of unity means that cases are no more likely to be exposed to the risk factor than controls. From Table 9.4 the odds ratio for contraceptive users and breast cancer patients is OR= $(537 \times 622)/(554 \times 639)$ = 0.94, indicating that breast cancer patients are slightly less likely to be contraceptive users. Note that the odds ratio can also be written $(a/b)/(c/d)$, i.e. having defined the cases and controls, it is the ratio of the odds of a woman selected from the study being a case given that she has used contraceptives to the odds of her being a case given that she never used contraceptives.

A method for calculating a 95% confidence interval for the true odds ratio is given in Appendix A13. For the odds ratio of oral contraceptives and breast cancer the confidence interval is 0.80 to 1.10. This confidence interval includes an OR equal to 1, implying that the hypothesis that the risk of breast cancer is not affected by oral contraceptive usage is consistent with the data. Note that the confidence interval in this case is asymmetric, with a shorter distance from the lower limit to the estimate of 0.94 than from the estimate to the upper limit.

(b) Matched studies

In some case-control studies each case is matched on an individual basis with a particular control. In this situation the analysis should take matching into account. The notation for a matched case-control study is given in Table 9.5.

In this situation each case/control pair is classified by exposure of the case and control. An important point here is that the concordant pairs, i.e. situations where the case and control are either both exposed or both not exposed, tell us

Table 9.5 Notation for a matched case-control study

		Controls		
		Exposed	Not exposed	Total
Cases	Exposed	e	f	a
	Not exposed	g	h	c
	Total	b	d	n

nothing about the risk of exposure separately for cases or controls. Consider a situation where it was required to discriminate between two students in tests which resulted in either a simple pass or fail. If the students are given a variety of tests, in some they will both pass and in some they will both fail. However, it is only by the tests where one student passes and the other fails, that a decision as to who is better can be given.

The odds ratio for a matched case-control study is given by f/g.

Example from the literature

Consider the study of testicular cancer by Brown, Pottern and Hoover (1987) and described in Sections 2.7 and 6.7. They conducted a matched case-control study, and one of the questions asked of both cases and controls was whether or not their testes were descended at birth. Part of the results of their study is given in Table 6.4.

The odds ratio for testicular cancer for subjects who had undescended testes is given by OR= 11/3 = 3.7. A 95% confidence interval was given by the authors as 0.9 to 10.4, which includes 1, and so there is not enough evidence to conclude that undescended testes are a risk factor for testicular cancer.

(c) Analysis by matching?

In many case-control studies matching is used not to control for important clinical factors that might produce bias, but merely as a convenient criterion for choosing controls. Thus for example, a control is often chosen to be of the same sex, of a similar age and with the same physician as the case. The question then arises whether one should take the matching into account in the analysis. The general rule is that the analysis should reflect the design. However, a matched analysis can be difficult to carry out and difficult to report. Feinstein (1987) gives a useful discussion of the issues involved. He shows that the matched and unmatched analyses will give similar results if, in the notation of Table 9.5, $f \times g$ is close to $e \times h$.

(d) Odds ratio and relative risk

By analogy with cohort studies one might argue that in a case-control study using the notation of Table 9.3, of those exposed, a proportion $a/(a+b)$ have the disease and of those not exposed, $c/(c+d)$ have the disease. Thus the relative risk is $a(c+d)/\{c(a+b)\}$. Such an argument is *incorrect*. To illustrate this consider the situation if one took twice as many controls. In general this would double both b and d, and so the relative risk would now appear to be $a(c+2d)/\{c(a+2b)\}$, which in most cases would be different from the previous estimate. Obviously, one would not expect to change the relative risk simply by increasing the number of controls and so the estimate must be erroneous. Note, however, that in a case-control study, if the number of controls is doubled the estimate of the odds ratio is not changed since both the numerator and the denominator of the expression are doubled.

The odds ratio gives a reasonable estimate of the relative risk when:

(1) The proportion of subjects classified with the disease is small.
(2) The cases and controls are random samples from the same relevant population group.

In many other situations, however, when these criteria are not strictly true, it has been found that the odds ratio estimated from a case-control study well approximates the relative risk of a cohort study conducted subsequently and thus results obtained from case-control studies are considered very valuable.

9.5 STANDARDISATION

The crude mortality rate for Chile in 1981 was 6.2 deaths per thousand per year, whereas that for the England and Wales for the same period was 11.8. Are we to infer that Chileans are much healthier than the English and Welsh? The important point here is that on average the Chileans are much younger than the English and Welsh, and young people of any nationality will have a lower mortality than old people. Thus we need to allow for the different age distributions of the two countries if we are to make comparisons.

Example from the literature

Beral, Fraser and Chilvers (1978) compared the mortality from ovarian cancer for different countries. They showed that the ovarian cancer rates appear to decrease with increasing completed family size.

An initial analysis might be to divide the number of cases of ovarian cancer for each country by the number of women for a particular year and compare proportions as described in Chapter 6. However, this approach ignores the fact that different countries have different age patterns. It is a well-known fact that cancer mortality is higher in older age groups and thus countries with older populations are likely to have more cancer deaths. We could compare age-specific rates but the difficulty here is that we would have to make as many comparisons as we have age groups.

There are two methods to standardise mortality rates of a target population for age. *Direct standardisation* calculates the age-specific rates in the target population and asks how many deaths would we expect in a standard population, that is, one with a fixed or defined age distribution, if these rates applied. The difficulty here is that if the target population is small the age-specific rates are not estimated very accurately and in fact one does not often see the method in the literature often. *Indirect standardisation* uses fixed or defined age-specific rates and asks how many deaths would be expected in the target population if these rates were to apply.

To standardise the mortality rate of a target population the following are required:

(1) A reference population with age-specific rates for the disease in question.
(2) The number of deaths in the target population over the period of interest. Note that the ages of subjects who die in the target population are not required.
(3) A census of the target population during the period referred to in (2) to provide counts specified by age group.

From the reference population rates and the age distribution of the target population we can calculate the number of deaths expected in the target population if the reference population rates had applied.

The *standardised mortality ratio* (SMR) for a defined target population and period is the ratio of the observed numbers of deaths in that area and period divided by the number expected if some standard age-specific mortality rates had prevailed. The ratio is usually multiplied by 100 so that if the number of deaths in the target population is exactly that predicted by the standard, the SMR will be 100. The method of calculating the SMR is described in Appendix A14.

Beral *et al.* (1978) used the age-specific rates for ovarian cancer for England and Wales as the reference population. The SMR for Chile for ovarian cancer was found to be 49 with an approximate standard error of 5.6. Thus the 95% confidence interval is given by

$$\text{SMR} - 1.96 \times \text{SE(SMR)} \quad \text{to} \quad \text{SMR} + 1.96 \times \text{SE(SMR)}$$

which is 38 to 60. Since this does not include 100 we conclude that the mortality from ovarian cancer in Chile is significantly lower than that in England and Wales, allowing for age.

SMRs can be calculated for a variety of definable groups and one often sees them quoted by occupation, social class, and region of a country. Care is needed to ensure that the numerator of the ratio (the deaths) actually refers to the same group as the denominator. For example, most people retire before they die, and usually their past occupation is obtained from the death certificate. Thus the deaths will refer to an occupational group in the past. However, it may be very difficult to determine the numbers 'at risk' in the past, that is people who did specific jobs during a given period. For example, if we suspect coal mining to be associated with gastric cancer, we could examine all death certificates in a specified area for mention of mining as a past occupation. However, in order to calculate death rates we would need to know the number of people employed as miners in the area for (say) 50 years in the past. A useful statistic to quote in these circumstances is the *proportional mortality ratio*, that is the number of deaths due to a particular cause divided by the total number of deaths.

The statistical model underlying the usefulness of SMRs is known as *proportional hazards*. Essentially this requires the relative risk of disease in the target population compared with the standard to be the same for each age group. If one age group in the target population were particularly at risk, then the SMR would tend to attenuate the affect, and the age-specific rates should be given.

9.6 ASSOCIATION AND CAUSALITY

Once an association between a risk factor and disease has been identified, a number of questions should be asked to try and strengthen the argument that the relationship is causal.

(1) *Consistency.* Have other investigators and other studies in different populations led to similar conclusions?
(2) *Plausibility.* Are the results biologically plausible? For example, if a risk factor is associated with cancer, are there known carcinogens in the risk factor?
(3) *Dose–response.* Are subjects with a heavy exposure to the risk factor at greater risk of disease than those with only slight exposure?
(4) *Temporality.* Does the disease incidence in a population increase or decrease following increasing or decreasing exposure to a risk factor? For example, lung cancer in women is increasing some years after the numbers of women taking up smoking increased.
(5) *Strength of the relationship.* A large relative risk may be more convincing than a small one (even if the latter is statistically significant). The difficulty with statistical significance is that it is a function of the sample size as well as the size of any possible effect. In an exercise that compares a large number of large groups some statistically significant differences are bound to occur.

9.7 POINTS WHEN READING THE LITERATURE

(1) In a cohort study, have a large percentage of the cohort been followed up, and have those lost to follow-up been described by their measurements at the start of the study?
(2) How has the cohort been selected? Is the method of selection likely to influence the variables that are measured?
(3) In a case-control study, are the cases likely to be typical of people with the disease?
(4) In a matched case-control study, has allowance been made for matching in the analysis?
(5) When an SMR is quoted, how has the population been defined? Does the numerator (the deaths) refer to the same population as the denominator?

Chapter 10

Common pitfalls in medical statistics

Summary

Some common errors found in the medical literature are described. They comprise problems in using the t-test, method comparison studies and repeated measure studies, plotting the change of a variable in time against the initial value, and confusing statistical and clinical significance.

10.1 INTRODUCTION

Many statistical errors in the medical literature might be described as venial, such as using a t-test when it is dubious that the data are Normally distributed, or failing to provide enough information for the reader to discover exactly how a test was carried out. There are frequent examples of poor presentation, or of presentation in the Abstract of results irrelevant to the problem being tackled by the paper. These errors do not usually destroy a paper's total credibility, they merely detract from its quality and serve to irritate the reader. However, some errors stem from a fundamental misunderstanding of the underlying reasoning in statistics, and these can produce spurious or incorrect analyses. It is to such errors that this chapter is addressed.

10.2 USING THE t-TEST

We give a fictitious example, which is based, however, on a number of published accounts. Thirty patients with chronic osteoarthritis were entered into a randomised double-blind two-group trial that compared a non-steroidal anti-inflammatory drug (NSAID) with a placebo. The trial period was one month. Table 10.1 summarises the change in the visual

Table 10.1 Results of two-group trial of an NSAID

Observation	Placebo		NSAID			
Number of patients (n)	15		15			
	Mean	SD	Mean	SD	t	p
Change in VAS (cm)	1.5	2.0	3.5	2.5	2.41	0.02
Number of tablets of paracetemol	20.1	19.7	15.1	14.7	0.79	NS
Haemoglobin (g/dl)	13.2	1.00	12.5	1.10	1.82	NS

analogue scale (VAS) rating for pain, the number of tablets of paracetamol taken during the study and the haemoglobin levels at the end of the study.

The first problem encountered with this table is that the degrees of freedom for the t-statistic are not given. If it is a straightforward two-sample t-test then they can be assumed to be $2n - 2 = 28$. However, it is possible that the data are paired in some way, and a paired test used, in which case df= $n - 1 = 14$; or the results come from an adjusted comparison, using multiple regression as described in Chapter 7. In both such cases the degrees of freedom will be less than the presumed 28. Of course, some clue to which is appropriate may be given in the supporting text.

The second problem is that the comparison of interest is the difference in response between the NSAID and placebo, together with an estimate of variability, and yet this comparison is not given. Two extra columns should therefore be added to Table 10.1. The first column would give the mean difference in the observations between placebo and NSAID, and the second a measure of the precision of this estimate, such as a 95% confidence interval.

From the data it can be seen that for both the change in VAS and the number of tablets taken, the standard deviations in each treatment group are of the same size as the mean. Since a change in VAS can be either positive or negative, this need not be a problem. However, the number of tablets taken must be zero or a positive number, and so the large standard deviation indicates that these data must be markedly skewed. This calls into question the validity of the use of the t-test on data which are non-Normal. Either a transformation of the original data or perhaps the non-parametric Mann–Whitney test as described in the Appendix A10 would be more appropriate.

For the number of tablets of paracetamol and haemoglobin the table gives p = NS. The abbreviation means 'not significant' and is usually taken to mean $p > 0.05$, but the notation is non-standard and should be avoided. Its use gives no indication of how close to $p = 0.05$ the results are. For the number of tablets of paracetamol taken, if df = 28 then from Table T2 $p > 0.10$ (exact value from Lindley and Scott, 1984 is $p = 0.42$) and for haemoglobin $0.05 < p < 0.10$ (exact value p = 0.08). Both are larger than the conventional value of 0.05 for formal statistical significance. However, it would be wrong to assert from this that the NSAID had no effect on haemoglobin. There is a difference in the means of 0.7 g/dl in the two groups at the end of the trial. The 95% confidence interval for the difference is −0.09 to 1.49 g/dl, indicating the possibility of the existence of quite a large effect of the NSAID on haemoglobin.

10.3 COMPARISON OF METHODS

Example from the literature

Figure 10.1 displays the results of a study discussed by Campbell and Williams (1989) in which 70 subjects had their FEV$_1$ measured by using a Respiradyne spirometer and a Vitalograph spirometer.

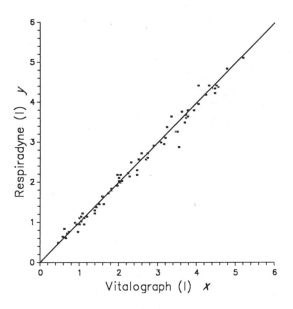

Figure 10.1   FEV$_1$ in 70 subjects by two different spirometers with the line of equality

A common method of analysis is first to calculate the correlation coefficient between the two sets of readings and then calculate a significance level on the null hypothesis of no association. Bland and Altman (1986) argue that this analysis is inappropriate for a number of reasons:

(i) The correlation coefficient is a measure of association. What is required here is a measure of agreement. We will have perfect correlation if the observations lie on any straight line, but perfect agreement only if the points lie on the line of equality.

(ii) The correlation coefficient observed depends on the range of measurements used. As discussed in Chapter 7, one can increase the correlation coefficient by choosing widely spaced observations. Since investigators usually compare two methods over the whole range of likely values, a good correlation is almost guaranteed.

(iii) Because of (ii), data which have an apparently high correlation can, for individual subjects, show very poor agreement between the methods of measurement.

(iv) The test of significance is not relevant since it would be very ·surprising if two methods designed to measure the same thing were not related.

Bland and Altman recommend an alternative approach. As an initial step one should plot the data as in Figure 10.1, but omit the calculation of a regression line and the corresponding test of significance. They argue that since most of the data will cluster about the line of equality, it can be difficult to assess differences between methods. The next step is to plot the paired difference between the two observations on each subject against the mean of these two readings, as shown in Figure 10.2 .

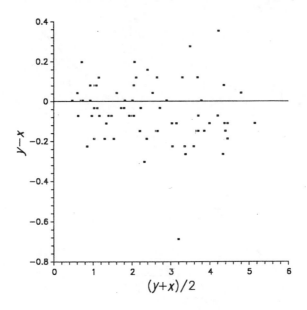

Figure 10.2   Scatter diagram of difference between methods against mean of both for data of Figure 10.1

It can be seen that there is no obvious relation between the difference and the mean. As a consequence the lack of agreement can be estimated by the mean difference, $\bar{d}$, which provides an estimate of the *bias*. For the FEV_1 data the mean difference $\bar{d} = 0.06$ l/sec and $SD(d) = s = 0.15$ l/sec. Bland and Altman suggest using the interval $\bar{d} - 2s$ to $\bar{d} + 2s$ as the 'limits of agreement'. For the FEV_1 data we get that the 'limits of agreement' are -0.24 to 0.36 l/sec. Thus one spirometer could give a reading as much as 0.36 l/sec above the other or 0.24 l/sec below it. Whether this is acceptable agreement needs to be judged from a clinical viewpoint. A test of significance of the correlation coefficient is not the appropriate criterion.

Another useful feature of the plot in Figure 10.2 is that the outlier becomes immediately apparent, but is not particularly prominent in Figure 10.1. If an outlier is present it is good practice to check the results for this subject. Perhaps there has been a mistake entering the data, and if necessary it could be that that subject is excluded from the calculations for the limits of agreement.

10.4 PLOTTING CHANGE AGAINST INITIAL VALUE

Example from the literature

Table 10.2 gives the birthweight and weight at one month of 20 babies randomly selected from a larger study carried out in Southampton by Campbell, Lewry and Wailoo (1988).

Table 10.2   Birth and one month weight of 10 babies (grams)

Birth-weight	Month weight	Weight gain (month − birth)	Mean (month + birth)/2
3888	4685	787	4286
3643	4019	375	3831
4065	4576	512	4320
3292	5317	2025	4304
2997	5492	2495	4244
4369	3700	−669	4035
2653	4199	1546	3426
2566	3854	1288	3210
4202	4293	91	4247
4219	4569	350	4394

One common question is of the form, 'Do lighter babies have a different rate of growth early in life?' A typical method of tackling this is to plot the change in weight against the birthweight as shown in Figure 10.3.

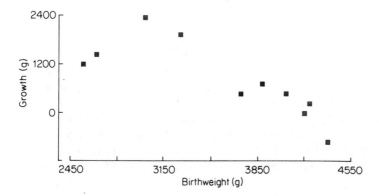

Figure 10.3   Growth of 10 babies in one month against birthweight

It would appear from the figure that smaller babies grow fastest, and indeed the correlation between birthweight and weight gain is $r = -0.79$, which has df = 8 and $p = 0.007$ by the test described in Appendix A11.

The problem here is the test of statistical significance. If we took any two sets of random numbers A and B and plotted $B - A$ on the y-axis against A on the x-axis, we will observe a negative association. This is because we have $-A$ in the y term and $+A$ in the x term. As a consequence we are guaranteed a negative correlation. This makes the test of significance for an association between a change and the initial value invalid.

Provided that the two sets of data have approximately the same variability a valid test of significance can be provided by correlating $(A - B)$ with $(A + B)/2$. Figure 10.4 shows weight gain plotted against the mean of birth and one-month weights.

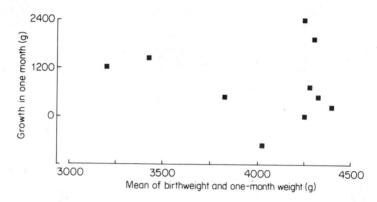

Figure 10.4   Weight gain of 10 babies in one month against the mean of birth and month weight

The corresponding correlation coefficient is $r = -0.13$ and with df $= 8$ this yields $p = 0.70$ (Appendix A11). The evidence for a relationship is much weaker using this approach.

Example from the literature

Findlay *et al.* (1987) give a graph showing the change in fasting serum cholesterol in 33 men after 30 weeks of training against their initial cholesterol level (Figure 10.5).

The correlation of $r = -0.57$ suggests that those with high initial levels changed the most. However, the correlation of the change with the mean of the initial and final levels is $r = 0.28$, df $= 31$ and $p = 0.11$. This implies that the association could well have arisen by chance, although if any relationship does exist it is more likely to be positive!

10.5 REPEATED MEASURES

A *regular design* used in the collection of clinical data is one in which a subject receives a treatment and then a response is measured on several occasions over a period of time.

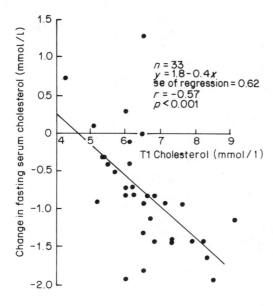

Figure 10.5   Change in fasting serum cholesterol concentrations after 30 weeks of training (after Findlay *et al.*, 1987, with permission)

Example from the literature

Figure 10.6 shows a graph of some results obtained in a recent study. The metabolic rate was measured over a two-hour period in 7 women following a test meal. The study was repeated at 12–15, 25–28 and 34–36 weeks of pregnancy. The corresponding values in the same women following lactation were used as controls.

The numerous significance tests would appear to imply, for example, that the metabolic rate 60 minutes after ingesting a meal was not significantly different from control, but that it was significantly different at 45 and 75 minutes after ingesting a meal, at 25–28 weeks.

(a) Invalid approaches

(1) The implication of the error bars in the graphs is that the true curve could be plausibly drawn through any point that did not take it outside the ranges shown. This is not true for several separate reasons. Since the error bars are in fact 68% confidence intervals (one standard error either side of the mean), then crudely there is a 68% chance that the true mean is within the limit. If there were ten independent observations, then the chances of the true line passing through each set of intervals is $0.68^{10} = 0.02$, which is very unlikely. However, the observations are certainly not independent, in which case this calculation only gives a guide to the true probability that the curve passes through all the intervals. It does suggest, however, that this probability is likely to be small.

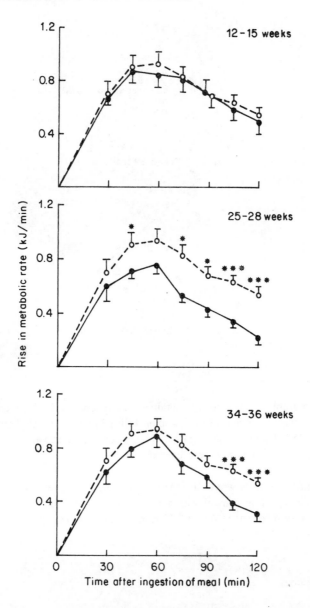

Figure 10.6 Rise in metabolic rate in response to test meal. Subjects after lactation (dotted line) and at 12–15, 25–28, and 34–36 weeks of pregnancy (solid line). Points are means. Bars are SEM. *$p<0.05$; ***$p<0.01$

(2) The average curve calculated from a set of individual curves may differ markedly from the shape of the individual curves. Three response curves are shown in Figure 10.7, together with their average. The individual responses are simply a sudden change from one level to another but these occur at different times for the three subjects. The average response gives the impression of a gradual change.

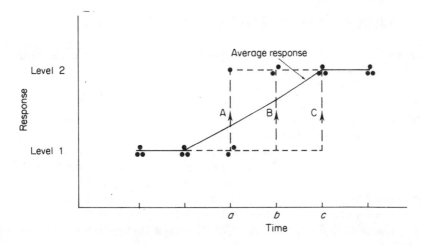

Figure 10.7 Response curves from three individuals and their average response at each time point. The three subjects change from level 1 to level 2 at times a, b, c respectively

(3) Often the purpose of the significance test is to ask the question, 'when does the response under one treatment differ from the response under another?' or 'when does the response differ from baseline?' It is a strange logic that perceives the difference between two continuous variables changing from not significantly different to significantly different between two adjacent time points. In practice measurements rarely jump suddenly from one level to another, but do so smoothly.

(b) Valid approaches

Having plotted the individual response curves, the usual approach is to try to find a small number of statistics that effectively summarise the data. For example in Figure 10.7, each individual can be summarised by the time at which they change. In Figure 10.6 the area under the curve from 0 to 120 minutes will effectively summarise the change in metabolic rate over the period.

Many repeated measure curves can be summarised by one or more of the following statistics:

(i) the area under the curve,
(ii) the maximum (or minimum) value achieved,
(iii) the time taken to reach the maximum (or minimum),
(iv) the slope of the line.

These statistics can then be used in an analysis as if they were raw observations; for example, one could compare the area under the metabolic rate curve for the four periods of Figure 10.6. In general, the analysis of repeated measures is quite tricky, and a statistician should be consulted early in the process.

The hazards of the analysis of repeated measures data are well described by Oldham (1968).

10.6 CLINICAL AND STATISTICAL SIGNIFICANCE

There are two aspects to consider, depending on whether or not the result under consideration is statistically significant.

(1) Given a large enough study, even small differences can become statistically significant.Thus in a clinical trial of two hypotensive agents, with 500 subjects on each treatment, one treatment reduced blood pressure on average by 30 mmHg and the other by 32 mmHg . Suppose the pooled standard deviation was 15.5 mmHg , then the two-sample z-test, which can be used since the samples are very large (Appendix A3), gives $z = 2.04$, $p = 0.04$. This is a statistically significant result which may be quoted in the Abstract as 'A was significantly better than B, $p = 0.04$', without any mention that it was a mere 2 mmHg better. Such a small difference, is of no importance to individual patients. Thus the result is statistically significant but not clinically important.

(2) On the other hand, given a small study, quite large differences fail to be statistically significant. For example, in a clinical trial of a placebo versus a hypotensive agent, each with 10 patients per group, the change in blood pressure for the placebo was 17 mmHg and for the hypotensive drug it was 30 mmHg. If the pooled standard deviation were 15.5 mmHg, by the two-sample t-test (Appendix A4) $t = 1.9$, df = 18 and $p = 0.06$. This fails to reach the conventional 5% significance level. However, the potential benefit from an additional reduction in blood pressure of 13 mmHg is substantial and so the result should not be ignored. It would be misleading to state in the Abstract 'There was no significant difference between drug A and placebo', and it would be better to quote the result achieved, 13 mmHg, together with a 95% confidence interval -2 to 28 mmHg.

10.7 EXPLORATORY DATA ANALYSIS AND 'FISHING EXPEDITIONS'

There is an important distinction to be made between studies that test well-defined hypotheses and studies where the investigator does not specify the hypotheses in advance. It is human nature to wish to collect as much data as possible on subjects entered in a study and having collected the data it is incumbent on the investigator to analyse it all to see if new and unsuspected relationships are revealed.

In these circumstances it is important, *a priori*, to separate out the main hypothesis (to be tested) and subsidiary hypotheses (to be explored) . During these so-called 'fishing expeditions' or 'data-dredging exercises' the notion of statistical significance as discussed in Chapter 6 plays no part at all. It can be used only as a guide to the relative importance of different results. Subsidiary hypotheses that are statistically significant should be presented in an exploratory manner, as results needing further testing with other studies. For clinical trials, this is particularly the case for sub-group analysis. Doctors are always interested to see if a particular treatment only works for a particular category of patient. The difficulty is that the sub-group is not usually specified in advance. Results of sub-group analysis, where the subgroups are discovered during the data processing, should always be treated with caution until confirmed by other studies.

If the data set is large, a different approach to 'fishing' is to divide it into two sets. One set is used for the exploratory analysis. This then generates the hypotheses that can be tested in the second set of data.

10.8 POINTS WHEN READING THE LITERATURE

(1) Are the distributional assumptions underlying parametric tests such as the t-test satisfied ? Is there any way of finding out?
(2) If a correlation coefficient is tested for significance, is the null hypothesis of zero correlation a sensible one?
(3) Is the study a repeated measures type? If so, beware!
(4) Are the results clinically significant as well as statistically significant? If the results are statistically not significant, is equivalence between groups being claimed? If the result is statistically significant, what is the size of the effect?
(5) Have a large number of tests been carried out that have not been reported? Were the hypotheses generated by an exploration of the data set, and then confirmed using the same data set?

Appendix I

Techniques

This appendix contains a brief description, with a worked example, of each of the commonly used statistical techniques. Where possible, the reader is encouraged to use a computer to process the results. In this way the data have to be entered only once, and the computations will be free of arithmetical mistakes. Good statistical packages are commercially available and these should be used in preference to 'home-produced' programs.

A1 NOTATION AND HINTS ON CALCULATION

We use the 'sigma' notation so that if we have n observations $x_1, x_2, \ldots, x_n$ then we will write Σx for

$$x_1 + x_2 + \ldots + x_n \quad \text{or} \quad \sum_{i=1}^{n} x_i$$

We often have to calculate quantities such as

$$\sum (x - \bar{x})^2 = (x_1 - \bar{x})^2 + (x_2 - \bar{x})^2 + \ldots + (x_n - \bar{x})^2$$

or, given a second set of observations $y_1, y_2, \ldots, y_n$,

$$\sum (x - \bar{x})(y - \bar{y}) = (x_1 - \bar{x})(y_1 - \bar{y}) + (x_2 - \bar{x})(y_2 - \bar{y}) + \ldots + (x_n - \bar{x})(y_n - \bar{y})$$

It can be shown that

$$\sum (x - \bar{x})^2 = \sum x^2 - \left(\sum x\right)^2 / n$$

and

$$\sum (x - \bar{x})(y - \bar{y}) = \sum xy - \left(\sum x \sum y\right)/n$$

The formulae on the right-hand side of the equation are easier to use with a calculator, and are often pre-programmed in electronic calculators with statistical functions. However, they should be used with care, because in certain circumstances, for example if the observations take large numerical values, then rounding errors can induce inaccuracies.

A2 CALCULATION OF MEAN AND STANDARD DEVIATION

Suppose a sample from a population consists of n observations x_1, x_2, ..., x_n. The sample mean, or average, is given by

$$\bar{x} = \sum x/n$$

The sample standard deviation is given by

$$s = \sqrt{\left\{\left[\sum (x - \bar{x})^2\right]/(n - 1)\right\}}$$

The *variance* is the square of the standard deviation. It is important to notice the divisor $n-1$ in the above formula. Some electronic calculators provide two options for calculating s which they denote by σ_n and σ_{n-1}. The n option effectively replaces $n - 1$ by n in the above expression for s. The σ_{n-1} option should always be chosen.

Example: Calculation of a mean and standard deviation

Table A1 FEV_1 from 5 asthmatic patients (litres/sec)

	x	$x - \bar{x}$	$(x - \bar{x})^2$	x^2
	1.5	−0.36	0.1296	2.25
	1.7	−0.16	0.0256	2.89
	2.1	0.24	0.0576	4.41
	1.6	−0.26	0.0676	2.56
	2.4	0.54	0.2916	5.76
Sum	9.3	0.00	0.5720	17.87

$\bar{x} = 9.3/5 = 1.86$, $s = \sqrt{(0.572/4)} = \sqrt{0.143} = 0.378$.

Note: 0.5720 is the sum of the third column in Table A1, or can be calculated by: $17.87 - (9.3)^2/5 = 0.5720$.

A3 TWO-SAMPLE z-TEST

We wish to test the null hypothesis that the means from two independent samples are equal, when the samples are large.

Sample 1: number of subjects n_1, mean $\bar{x}_1$, standard deviation s_1.
Sample 2: number of subjects n_2, mean $\bar{x}_2$, standard deviation s_2.

Assumptions
(1) Data are plausibly Normally distributed.
(2) Data are independent.
(3) Samples are large ($n_1 > 30$, $n_2 > 30$).

Calculate the standard error of the difference between the means as

$$SE(\bar{x}_1 - \bar{x}_2) = \sqrt{\left\{ \frac{s_1^2}{n_1} + \frac{s_2^2}{n_2} \right\}}$$

and

$$z = (\bar{x}_1 - \bar{x}_2)/SE(\bar{x}_1 - \bar{x}_2)$$

Under the null hypothesis, z is distributed approximately as a Normal distribution (Table T1), with mean zero, and standard deviation 1. A 95% confidence interval for the difference is

$$(\bar{x}_1 - \bar{x}_2) - 1.96\,SE(\bar{x}_1 - \bar{x}_2) \quad \text{to} \quad (\bar{x}_1 - \bar{x}_2) + 1.96\,SE(\bar{x}_1 - \bar{x}_2)$$

Example

Diabetics' systolic blood pressure: $n_1 = 100$, $\bar{x}_1 = 135$ mmHg, $s_1 = 10$ mmHg. ·
Controls' systolic blood pressure: $n_2 = 90$, $\bar{x}_2 = 125$ mmHg, $s_2 = 6$ mmHg.
$SE(\bar{x}_1 - \bar{x}_2) = 1.18$, $z = 8.47$.

From Table T1 we find that for $z = 3.09$, $p = 0.002$, and thus for $z = 8.47$, $p \ll 0.002$. A 95% confidence interval for the difference in blood pressure between the groups is $10 - 1.96 \times 1.18$ to $10 + 1.96 \times 1.18$, which is 7.68 to 12.32 mmHg.

A4 TWO-SAMPLE t-TEST

Suppose we wish to test the null hypothesis that the means from two independent samples are equal but the sample sizes are small.

Sample 1: number of subjects n_1, mean $\bar{x}_1$, standard deviation s_1.
Sample 2: number of subjects n_2, mean $\bar{x}_2$, standard deviation s_2.

Assumptions
(1) Data are plausibly Normally distributed.
(2) Data are independent.
(3) Standard deviations are equal.

Calculate a pooled standard deviation by

$$s_p = \sqrt{\left\{\frac{(n_1 - 1)s_1^2 + (n_2 - 1)s_2^2}{n_1 + n_2 - 2}\right\}}$$

The standard error of the difference is

$$SE(\bar{x}_1 - \bar{x}_2) = s_p\sqrt{\left\{\frac{1}{n_1} + \frac{1}{n_2}\right\}}$$

and

$$t = (\bar{x}_1 - \bar{x}_2)/SE(\bar{x}_1 - \bar{x}_2)$$

Under the null hypothesis, this is distributed as Student's *t*-distribution (Table T2) with $n_1 + n_2 - 2$ degrees of freedom.
    A 95% confidence interval for the difference with $n_1 + n_2 - 2$ degrees of freedom is

$$(\bar{x}_1 - \bar{x}_2) - t_{0.05} \times SE(\bar{x}_1 - \bar{x}_2) \quad \text{to} \quad (\bar{x}_1 - \bar{x}_2) + t_{0.05} \times SE(\bar{x}_1 - \bar{x}_2)$$

Example

Asthmatics' FEV_1: $n_1 = 5$, $\bar{x}_1 = 1.86$, $s_1 = 0.378$.
Controls' FEV_1 : $n_2 = 6$, $\bar{x}_2 = 2.51$, $s_2 = 0.210$.
Then $s_p = 0.297$, $SE(\bar{x}_1 - \bar{x}_2) = 0.180$, $t = 0.65/0.180 = 3.62$, df= $5 + 6 - 2 = 9$.

    From Table T2, with 9 degrees of freedom, $t_{0.01} = 3.25$, therefore $p < 0.01$.
A 95% confidence interval for the difference is given by $0.65 - 2.201 \times 0.180$ to
$0.65 + 2.201 \times 0.180$, which is 0.25 to 1.05 litres/sec.

A5 PAIRED *t*-TEST

Let $x_{11}, x_{12}, \ldots, x_{1n}$ be the observations in group 1 and $x_{21}, x_{22}, \ldots, x_{2n}$ be the corresponding observations in group 2 such that x_{1i} is paired with x_{2i}. Calculate $d_i = x_{1i} - x_{2i}$, $i = 1, \ldots, n$.

Assumptions
(1) The d_i's are plausibly Normally distributed (note it is not essential for the original observations to be Normally distributed).
(2) The d_i's are independent of each other.

Calculate the mean $\bar{d}$, the standard deviation, s_d, of the differences d_i, the $SE(\bar{d}) = s_d/\sqrt{n}$ and finally $t = \bar{d}/SE(\bar{d})$. Under the null hypothesis, t is distributed as Student's t, with $n - 1$ degrees of freedom.

Example

Table A2 FEV_1 from 5 asthmatics, before and after use of a bronchodilator (litres/sec)

x_1	x_2	$d = x_1 - x_2$
1.5	1.7	−0.2
1.7	1.9	−0.2
2.1	2.2	−0.1
1.6	1.9	−0.3
2.4	2.4	0.0
Sum		−0.8

$\bar{d} = -0.8/5 = -0.16$, $s_d = 0.114$, $SE(\bar{d}) = 0.114/\sqrt{5} = 0.0510$, and $t = -0.16/0.0510 = -3.14$.

For comparison with the statistical tables ignore the minus sign. From Table T2 with df = 4 the tabulated values are $t_{0.04} = 3.007$, and $t_{0.03} = 3.319$, and therefore $0.03 < p < 0.04$.

The 95% confidence interval for the difference is given by $-0.16 - 2.776 \times 0.051$ to $-0.16 + 2.776 \times 0.114$ or -0.30 to -0.02 litres/sec.

A6 χ^2 TEST IN 2×2 TABLES

In an unmatched case-control study, a clinical trial or a cross-sectional survey, the analysis might involve a comparison in proportions; for example, proportion exposed to a hazard in cases and controls in a case control study, or proportion cured under treatments A and B in a clinical trial. The classifying variables are termed *factors* and in Table A3 they are labelled A and B.

Table A3   Notation for unmatched 2×2 table
Numbers of subjects classified by factors A and B

		Factor A		
		Present	Absent	Total
Factor B	Present	a	b	$a + b$
	Absent	c	d	$c + d$
Total		$a + c$	$b + d$	N

Factor A might represent treatment or control, and factor B whether or not the subject was cured.

It is a convenient fact in statistics that we can use the χ^2 test, both for testing the significance of differences in proportions from zero, and for the significance of an odds ratios or a relative risk from unity.

The general form of a χ^2 test is to calculate the values expected in the four cells of the table assuming the null hypothesis is true. For row i and column j of the table, if R_i is the row total, C_j the column total and N the overall total, the expected value for that particular cell is $E_{ij} = C_j \times R_i/N$. Thus the expected value for the numbers of subjects with both factor A and factor B present is

$$E_{11} = \frac{(a + c)(a + b)}{N}$$

The χ^2 test is calculated from

$$\chi^2 = \sum (O - E)^2/E$$

using the O's and respective E's from the four cells of the table. In general, the application of *Yates' correction* to this calculation is recommended. In this case the calculation is

$$\chi^2 = \sum (|O - E| - \tfrac{1}{2})^2/E$$

where the modulus sign $|\ |$ means take the positive value. For ease of calculation this can be shown to be equivalent to

$$\chi_c^{\ 2} = \frac{(|ad - bc| - \tfrac{1}{2}N)^2 N}{(a + b)(a + c)(b + d)(c + d)}$$

Under the null hypothesis that the two factors are independent, $\chi_c^{\ 2}$ has a chi-squared distribution with 1 degree of freedom.

Example

In a clinical trial of aspirin versus placebo in the treatment of headache the results were as shown in Table A4.

Table A4 Results of trial on headache and aspirin

	No headache	Headache	Total	Proportion
Aspirin	70	30	100	0.70
Placebo	55	55	110	0.50
Total	125	85	210	

We wish to examine whether the difference in those cured with aspirin (70%) and placebo (50%) could have arisen by chance.

The expected values are given in Table A5.

Table A5 Expected values for Table A4

	No headache	Headache	Total
Aspirin	59.5	40.5	100
Placebo	65.5	44.5	100
Total	125	85	210

Thus

$$\chi_c^2 = \frac{(|70 - 59.5| - \frac{1}{2})^2}{59.5} + \frac{(|30 - 40.5| - \frac{1}{2})^2}{40.5} + \frac{(|55 - 65.5| - \frac{1}{2})^2}{65.5}$$

$$+ \frac{(|55 - 44.5| - \frac{1}{2})^2}{44.5} = 7.92$$

Alternatively,

$$\chi_c^2 = \frac{(|70 \times 55 - 30 \times 55| - 105)^2 \times 210}{100 \times 110 \times 125 \times 85} = 7.89$$

(The slight discrepancy arises because the expected values are rounded to one decimal place.) Table T3 with 1 degree of freedom gives $\chi^2_{0.01} = 6.63$ and $\chi^2_{0.001} = 10.83$, and therefore $0.001 < p < 0.01$.

An approximate 95% confidence interval for the true difference in proportions can be calculated as follows. First calculate $p_1 = a/(a+b)$ and $p_2 = c/(c+d)$. The standard error for the difference $p_1 - p_2$ is given by

$$SE(p_1 - p_2) = \sqrt{\left\{ \frac{p_1(1 - p_1)}{a + b} + \frac{p_2(1 - p_2)}{c + d} \right\}}$$

The 95% confidence interval for the true difference in proportions is

$$(p_1 - p_2) - 1.96 \times SE(p_1 - p_2) \qquad to \qquad (p_1 - p_2) + 1.96 \times SE(p_1 - p_2)$$

The difference in proportions in Table A4 is $p_1 - p_2 = 0.20$, and $SE(p_1 - p_2) = 0.066$ and the approximate 95% confidence interval is $0.20 - 1.96 \times 0.066$ to $0.20 + 1.96 \times 0.066$, or 0.07 to 0.33.

A7 FISHER'S EXACT TEST FOR A 2×2 TABLE

If any expectation in a 2×2 table is less than about 5, the χ^2 test is inapplicable. Given the notation of Table A3 the probability of observing the particular table is

$$\frac{(a + b)!(c + d)!(a + c)!(b + d)!}{N!a!b!c!d!}$$

where the factorial $n!$ means $1 \times 2 \times 3 \times \ldots \times (n - 1) \times n$ and 0! and 1! are both taken to be unity. We next calculate the probability of other tables that can be identified that have the same marginal totals as the table giving the results of the study and also give as much or more evidence for an association between the factors. These probabilities are then summed and for a two-sided test we double the probability so obtained.

Example

Table A6 Deaths in 6 months after fractured neck of femur in a specialised orthopaedic ward (A) and a general ward (B)

(i)

		Ward		
		A	B	Total
Deaths	Yes	2	6	8
	No	18	14	32
Total		20	20	40

The probability of observing such a table, given the margins is

$$P(\text{i}) = \frac{8! \; 32! \; 20! \; 20!}{2! \; 6! \; 18! \; 14! \; 40!} = 0.095\,760$$

There are two rearrangements of the table which give as much or more evidence for the association. These are:

(ii)

	A	B	Total
Yes	1	7	8
No	19	13	32
Total	20	20	40

(iii)

	A	B	Total
Yes	0	8	8
No	20	12	32
Total	20	20	40

The probabilities associated with these tables are $P(\text{ii}) = 0.020\,160$ and $P(\text{iii}) = 0.001\,638$. Thus the total probability is $0.095\,760 + 0.020\,160 + 0.001\,638 = 0.117\,558$. For a two-sided test we double this to get $p = 0.24$. The confidence interval calculation in this situation is described, for example, in Gardner and Altman (1989).

A8 $r \times c$ TABLES

The 2×2 table is rather a special case. Consider counts in cells coming from a cross-classification of two factors, at least one of which has more than two levels.

Table A7 Notation for $r \times c$ tables

			Factor A level					
			1	2	3	...	r	Total
Factor B	Level	1	O_{11}	O_{12}	OO_{13}	...	O_{1r}	R_1
		2	O_{21}	O_{22}	O_{23}	...	O_{2r}	R_2
		3	.	.	.	...	.	.
		.	.	.	.	...	.	.
		c	O_{c1}	O_{c2}	O_{c3}	...	O_{cr}	R_c
	Total		C_1	C_2	C_3	...	C_r	N

Then the χ^2 statistic with $(r-1) \times (c-1)$ degrees of freedom uses the expected values $E_{ij} = C_j \times R_i/N$ corresponding to each O_{ij} in the expression.

$$\chi^2 = \sum (O - E)^2/E$$

The summation is over all the $c \times r$ cells of the table. This expression can be rewritten

$$\chi^2 = \sum \frac{O^2}{E} - N$$

which is easier for hand calculation.

It is important to remember that one does not use Yates's correction for contingency tables other than 2×2 tables.

Example

The data in Table A8 are on individuals with brain tumours, classified by tumour type and site.

Table A8 Results of study on brain tumour type and site

			Type		
		Benign	Malignant	Other	Total
	Frontal	23	9	6	38
Site	Temporal	21	4	3	28
	Other	34	24	17	75
		78	37	26	141

On the null hypothesis that the type of tumour is independent of the site, the expected number of subjects with benign tumours in the frontal lobes, for example, is $78 \times 38/141 = 21.02$. Computing the expected values for the whole table, $\chi^2 = 7.84$. There are $(3-1) \times (3-1) = 4$ degrees of freedom. From Table T3, $\chi^2_{0.05}$ with 4 degrees of freedom is 9.49, and $\chi^2_{0.1} = 7.78$, thus $0.05 < p < 0.10$.

Chi-Squared test for trend ($2 \times c$ table)

An important class of tables are $2 \times c$ tables, where the multi-level factor has ordered levels. For example, patients might score their pain on an integer scale from 1 to 5 on one of two treatments. In this case the χ^2 test is very inefficient, because it fails to take account of the ordering. In this case one should use the χ^2 test for trend. In this test one must assign scores to ordered outcome. So long as the scores reflect the ordering, the actual values affect the result little. Consider the notation in Table A9, which gives the results of a parallel clinical trial with ordered outcomes.

Table A9   Results of parallel clinical trial of two treatments

	Worse	Same	Outcome of trial Slightly better	Moderately better	Much better	Total
Treatment A (a_i)	11	53	42	27	11	144
Treatment B	1	13	16	15	7	52
Total (n_i)	12	66	58	42	18	196 (N)
$p_i = a_i/n_i$	0.0833	0.1970	0.2759	0.3571	0.3889	0.2653 ($\bar{p}$)
Score (x_i)	-2	-1	0	1	2	

With the notation given in Table A9, calculate

$$E = \sum n_i(p_i - \bar{p})(x_i - \bar{x}) = \sum a_i x_i - \left(\sum a_i\right)\left(\sum n_i x_i\right)/N$$

and

$$F = \sum n_i x^2_i - (n_i x_i)^2/N$$

Finally $\chi^2 = E^2/(F\,\bar{p}\,\bar{q})$ where $\bar{q} = 1 - \bar{p}$ has 1 df.

Thus from the Table A9 $E = -26 - 144 \times (-12)/196 = -17.18$, $F = 228 - (-12)^2/196 = 227.27$ and $\chi^2 = (-17.18)^2/(227.27 \times 0.2653 \times 0.7347) = 6.66$. From Table T3, with 1 df, we find $p = 0.01$.

The χ^2 test for trend is described by Armitage and Berry (1987, page 372). An alternative approach is to use the Mann–Whitney U test (with allowance for ties) described in Appendix A10.

A9 McNEMAR'S TEST

Although the calculations are the same for a case-control study or crossover trial, the arrangement of the table is somewhat different and so we give an example of each in Tables A10 and A11.

Table A10   Notation for McNemar's test (matched case-control study)

		Controls Exposed	Not exposed	Total
Cases	Exposed	e	f	$e + f$
	Not exposed	g	h	$g + h$
		$e + g$	$f + h$	n

Table A11   Notation for McNemar's test (crossover trial)

| | | Treatment A | | |
		Responded to treatment	Did not respond to treatment	Total
Treatment B	Responded to treatment	e	f	$e + f$
	Did not respond to treatment	g	h	$g + h$
	Total	$e + g$	$f + h$	n

Thus there are n pairs of subjects in the matched case-control study, and n subjects in the cross-over trial. In both cases calculate

$$\chi^2 = \frac{(f - g)^2}{f + g}$$

We recommend including Yates's correction for continuity, in which case the formula becomes

$$\chi_c^{\,2} = \frac{(|f - g| - 1)^2}{f + g}$$

In either case the test statistic is then compared with a χ^2 distribution with 1 df.

Example

In a clinical trial of two drugs A and B for arthritis, patients were given each drug in a randomised crossover study, and asked whether they were 'satisfied' or 'not satisfied' with the drug. The results are given in Table A12.

Table A12   Results of crossover trial of two drugs for arthritis

| | | Drug A | | |
		Satisfied	Not satisfied	Total
Drug B	Satisfied	150	20	170
	Not satisfied	30	50	80
Total		180	70	250

We calculate $\chi^2 = \dfrac{(|20 - 30| - 1)^2}{(20 + 30)} = \dfrac{81}{50} = 1.62.$

The tabulated value for χ^2 with 1 df is given from Table T3 as $\chi^2_{0.2} = 1.64$, hence $p \approx 0.2$.

Small samples

The exact test requires the calculation of $P = \frac{(f+g)!}{f!\,g!}\left(\frac{1}{2}\right)^{f+g}$ for the table observed and those indicating a stronger association with the same total $f + g$ of discordant pairs. These probabilities are then summed and for a two-sided test we double the probability so obtained.

Example

In the case-control of Brown, Pottern and Hoover (1987) the four tables for calculation are

(i)		(ii)		(iii)		(iv)	
4	11	4	12	4	13	4	14
3	241	2	241	1	241	0	241

giving $P(\mathrm{i}) = \dfrac{14!}{11!\,3!}\left(\dfrac{1}{2}\right)^{14} = 0.022\,217$

$P(\mathrm{ii}) = \dfrac{14!}{12!\,2!}\left(\dfrac{1}{2}\right)^{14} = 0.005\,554$

$P(\mathrm{iii}) = \dfrac{14!}{13!\,1!}\left(\dfrac{1}{2}\right)^{14} = 0.000\,854$

$P(\mathrm{iv}) = \dfrac{14!}{14!\,0!}\left(\dfrac{1}{2}\right)^{14} = 0.000\,061$

Thus the total probability is $0.028\,686$. For a two-sided test $p = 0.057$. This is very close to the value calculated in Section 6.7 using a χ^2 test with Yates's correction.

A10 NON-PARAMETRIC TESTS

If the data are clearly not Normally distributed, and there is no simple transformation to render it so, for example, if there are outliers in the data, then it is worth considering a nonparametric test.

(a) Mann–Whitney U test

If the data are from two independent groups of size n_1 and n_2 respectively and are at least ordinal, that is they can be ranked, then one can use the Mann–Whitney U test.

First combine the two groups and rank the entire data set. In the case of ties, that is two values that are equal, give the average rank to each. Sum the ranks for one of the groups. Let T be the sum of the ranks for the n_1 observations in this group. If there are no or only a few ties, calculate

$$z = \frac{T - n_1(n_1 + n_2 + 1)/2}{\sqrt{\{(n_1 n_2(n_1 + n_2 + 1)/12\}}}$$

On the null hypothesis that the two samples come from the same population, this z is approximately Normally distributed with mean zero and standard deviation 1, and can be referred to Table T1 to calculate a p-value.

Many textbooks give special tables for the Mann–Whitney U test, when sample sizes are small, that is when n_1 and n_2 are less than 20. However, the above expression is sufficiently accurate for most purposes. This formula is not accurate if there are many ties in the data. The reader is referred to Conover (1981) in such situations.

Example

After a randomised trial comparing aspirin with placebo for headache, 8 patients on aspirin and 10 on placebo rated their improvement on a 10 cm line, a measure of 0 indicating no improvement and one of 10 indicating very much better. The results are given in Table A13.

Table A13 Results of aspirin trial (VAS scale in centimetres to rate improvement of headache)

Aspirin	$n_1 = 8$:	7.5	8.3	9.1	6.2	5.4	8.3	6.5	8.4		
Placebo	$n_2 = 10$;	3.1	5.6	4.5	6.2	5.1	5.3	5.5	4.1	4.3	4.2

Order the 18 observations and assign ranks from smallest to largest below. The aspirin group observations are underlined in this ordering.

Observation	3.1	4.1	4.2	4.3	4.5	5.1	5.3	5.4	5.5
Rank	1	2	3	4	5	6	7	8	9

Observation	5.6	6.2	6.2	6.5	7.5	8.3	8.3	8.4	9.1
Rank	10	11.5	11.5	13	14	15	16	17	18

The sum of the ranks in the aspirin group gives $T = 112.5$, thus

$$z = \frac{112.5 - 8 \times 19/2}{\sqrt{\{8 \times 10 \times 19/12\}}} = 3.24$$

From Table T1 we find the smallest tabulated value of $z = 2.99$ corresponding to $\alpha = 0.0028$. Thus we know that $p < 0.003$ (to one significant figure).

(b) Wilcoxon signed-rank test

When the data are paired, for example in a matched case-control study, or a crossover trial, then the pairing should be taken into account in the analysis. The procedure is to subtract one member of the pair from the other, and then rank the resulting differences, but ignoring the respective plus or minus signs. Once the ranking is made, the signs are restored, so that the sum of the ranks associated with the plus sign gives T. We then compute

$$z = \frac{T - n(n + 1)/4}{\sqrt{\{n(n + 1)(2n + 1)/24\}}}$$

where n is the number of pairs.

We compare z to the tabulated Normal distribution in Table T1.

Example

Consider a matched case-control study of breast cancer and the oral contraceptive pill (OC). Ten women with breast cancer were matched with ten age, sex and social class controls, and the total duration of time they used the OC was noted. The results are given in Table A14.

Table A14 Duration of time using Oral Contraception (years)

Pair	1	2	3	4	5	6	7	8	9	10
Case	2.0	10.0	7.1	2.3	3.0	4.1	10.0	10.5	12.1	15.0
Control	1.5	9.1	8.1	1.5	3.1	5.2	1.0	9.6	7.6	9.0
Difference	0.5	0.9	−1.0	0.8	−0.1	−1.1	9.0	0.9	4.5	6.0
Ignoring signs	0.5	0.9	1.0	0.8	0.1	1.1	9.0	0.9	4.5	6.0
Ranks	2	4.5	6	3	1	7	10	4.5	8	9
Signed ranks	2	4.5	−6	3	−1	−7	10	4.5	8	9

Thus $T = 2 + 4.5 + 3 + 10 + 4.5 + 8 + 9 = 41$.

From the above formula we get

$$z = (41 - 27.5)/9.8 = 1.4.$$

From table T1 with $z = 1.4$ we get $p = 0.16$.

Methods for calculating confidence intervals associated with non-parametric tests are described by Campbell and Gardner (1988).

A11 CORRELATION COEFFICIENT

Given a set of pairs of observations (x_1, y_1), (x_2, y_2), ... , (x_n, y_n) the Pearson correlation coefficient is given by

$$r = \frac{\sum(x - \bar{x})(y - \bar{y})}{\sqrt{\{\sum(x - \bar{x})^2 \sum(y - \bar{y})^2\}}}$$

To test whether this is significantly different from zero, calculate

$$SE(r) = \sqrt{\{(1 - r^2)/(n - 2)\}} \text{ and } t = r/SE(r)$$

and compare this with the t-distribution of Table T2 with $n - 2$ degrees of freedom.

Example

Consider that the FVC was also measured in the asthmatic patients of Table A1, and the results given in Table A15.

Table A15   Relationship between FEV 1 and FVC in 5 asthmatics

	FEV$_1$ (y)	FVC (x)	xy	y^2	x^2
	1.5	2.0	3.00	2.25	4.00
	1.7	3.0	5.10	2.89	9.00
	2.1	2.9	6.09	4.41	8.41
	1.6	2.5	4.00	2.56	6.25
	2.4	3.0	7.20	5.76	9.00
Total	9.3	13.4	25.39	17.87	36.66

From the table, $n = 5$, $\bar{y} = 1.86$, $\bar{x} = 2.68$.

$$r = \frac{25.39 - 9.3 \times 13.4/5}{\sqrt{(17.87 - 9.32^2/5)(36.66 - 13.4^2/5)}} = \frac{0.466}{0.654} = 0.71$$

Thus $SE(r) = \sqrt{\{1 - 0.71^2)/3\}} = 0.41$ and $t = 0.71/0.41 = 1.73$.
  From Table T2, with df= $5 - 2 = 3$, $t_{0.1} = 0.10$, hence $p > 0.1$.

A12 LINEAR REGRESSION

Given a set of pairs of observations (x_1, y_1), (x_2, y_2), ..., (x_n, y_n) the regression coefficient of y given x is

$$b = \frac{\sum(x - \bar{x})(y - \bar{y})}{\sum(x - \bar{x})^2}$$

The intercept is estimated by $a = \bar{y} - b\bar{x}$.
  To test whether b is significantly different from zero, calculate

$$E = \sum(y - \bar{y})^2 - b^2 \sum(x - \bar{x})^2$$

$$F = (n - 2) \sum(x - \bar{x})^2$$

and

$$SE(b) = \sqrt{(E/F)}$$

Compare $t = b/\text{SE}(b)$ with the t-distribution of Table T2 with $n - 2$ degrees of freedom.

A 95% confidence interval for the slope, with $n - 2$ degrees of freedom is given by

$$b - t_{0.05}\text{SE}(b) \qquad \text{to} \qquad b + t_{0.05}\text{SE}(b).$$

Example

Table A16 Relationship between FEV_1 and height in five asthmatics

FEV$_1$ (l) (y)	Ht (cm) (x)	xy	y^2	x^2
1.5	160	240.0	2.25	25 600
1.7	170	289.0	2.89	28 900
2.1	173	363.3	4.41	29 929
1.6	165	264.0	2.56	27 225
2.4	175	420.0	5.76	30 625
9.3	843	1576.3	17.87	142 279

Thus $n = 5$, $\bar{y} = 1.86$, $\bar{x} = 168.6$, $\sum(y - \bar{y})^2 = \sum y^2 - n\bar{y}^2 = 0.572$, $\sum(x - \bar{x})^2 = \sum x^2 - n\bar{x}^2 = 149.2$, $\sum(x - \bar{x})(y - \bar{y}) = \sum xy - n\bar{x}\,\bar{y} = 8.32$, $b = 8.32/149.2 = 0.0558$ and $a = -7.54$. From these $E = 0.1074$, $F = 447.6$ and $\text{SE}(b) = \sqrt{(0.1074/447.6)} = 0.0155$.

Thus the regression line is estimated by $\text{FEV}_1 = -7.54 + 0.056 \times \text{Height}$. The formal test of significance of the regression coefficient requires $t = 0.056/0.0155 = 3.59$. We compare this with a t-distribution with df$= 5 - 2 = 3$. Use of Table T2 gives $p \approx 0.04$. The 95% confidence interval for the slope is given by $0.056 - 3.182 \times 0.0155$ to $0.056 + 3.182 \times 0.0155$, that is 0.007 to 0.105 litres/cm.

A13 CONFIDENCE INTERVAL FOR ODDS RATIO (OR) FROM AN UNMATCHED CASE-CONTROL STUDY

Using the notation of Table 9.4 the standard error of the log OR, in large samples, is given by

$$\text{SE}(\log \text{OR}) = \sqrt{\left\{\frac{1}{a} + \frac{1}{b} + \frac{1}{c} + \frac{1}{d}\right\}}$$

Thus for the data of Table 9.4

$$\text{SE}(\log \text{OR}) = \sqrt{\left\{\frac{1}{537} + \frac{1}{554} + \frac{1}{639} + \frac{1}{622}\right\}} = 0.083$$

In the example in Section 9.4, OR was calculated to be 0.94, so log OR is -0.06.

A 95% confidence interval for log OR is

$$\log OR - 1.96 \ SE(\log OR) \qquad \text{to} \qquad \log OR + 1.96 \ SE(\log OR)$$

This gives a confidence interval for log OR of -0.23 to 0.10. The corresponding 95% confidence interval for the OR is $e^{-0.23}$ to $e^{0.10}$, which is 0.80 to 1.10.

The reason for computing the standard error on the logarithmic scale is that this is more likely to be Normally distributed than the OR itself. It is important to note that when transformed back to the original scale, the confidence interval so obtained will be asymmetric about the OR. There will be a shorter distance from the lower confidence limit to the OR than from the OR to the upper confidence limit.

Further examples of this calculation, and that for a relative risk and an SMR (see below) are given by Morris and Gardner (1988).

A14 CALCULATION AND CONFIDENCE INTERVAL FOR AN SMR

The 1981 census of the City of Southampton, and a private census of Southampton University (staff and students) were used to obtain the age distribution of the two populations. The age-specific death rates for England and Wales in 1981 were also obtained and the results shown in Table A17.

Table A17 Population of the City of Southampton and the University and national age-specific death rates

Age group	City	University	Standard rates (per 1000)
0–4	25 000	—	0.8
5–14	40 000	—	0.4
15–24	55 000	7500	0.9
25–34	50 000	1500	1.0
35–44	42 000	200	2.3
45–54	27 000	150	7.1
55–64	17 000	70	20.0
65–74	10 000	10	52.0
75–84	5 000	—	120.0
85+	1 000	—	240.0
All ages	272 000	9430	

The observed number of deaths in the City in 1981 was 2200, and in the University was 6. We wish to compare the mortality of the City and the University.

To compute expected deaths, multiply the population by age-specific death rates, as in Table A18.

Table A18 Computing the expected deaths in the City and University of Southampton

Age group (1)	City (2)	University (3)	Rates (4)	Expected City $(2)\times(4)/1000$	Expected University $(3)\times(4)/1000$
0–4	25 000	—	0.8	20	—
5–14	40 000	—	0.4	16	—
15–24	55 000	7500	0.9	49.5	6.75
25–34	50 000	1500	1.0	50	1.50
35–44	42 000	200	2.3	96.6	0.46
45–54	27 000	150	7.1	191.7	1.07
55–64	17 000	70	20.0	340	1.40
65–74	10 000	10	52.0	520	0.52
75–84	5 000	—	120.0	600	—
85+	1 000	—	240.0	240	—
Total	272 000	9430		2123.8	11.70

The crude death rate are: City= 2200/72 000 = 8.1 deaths per 1000, and University= 6/9430 = 0.6 deaths per 1000.

The SMRs are: City= $100 \times O/E = 100 \times 2200/2123.8 = 103.6$ and for the University $100 \times 6/11.70 = 51.3$, where O and E are the corresponding numbers of observed and expected deaths.

Now approximately SE(SMR) = $\frac{\text{SMR}}{\sqrt{O}}$, thus for the City SE = $103.6/\sqrt{2200} = 2.21$ and the University SE = $51/\sqrt{6} = 20.8$.

The corresponding confidence intervals are:

City: $103.6 - 1.96 \times 2.2$ to $103.6 + 1.96 \times 2.2$ or 99.3 to 107.9
University: $51 - 1.96 \times 20.8$ to $51 + 1.96 \times 20.8$ or 10.2 to 91.8

A15 SAMPLE SIZE CALCULATIONS

As described in Chapters 1 and 8, to compute sample sizes we need to specify a significance level α and a power $1 - \beta$. The calculations depend on a function $(z_\alpha + z_\beta)^2$, where z_α and z_β are the ordinates for the normal distribution (Table T1). Some convenient values for a two-sided significance level of 5% are given in Table A19.

Table A19 Table to assist in sample size calculations, $\alpha = 0.05$

β	Power $(1 - \beta)$	z_β	z_α	$(z_\alpha + z_\beta)^2$
0.50	0.50	0.000	1.960	3.842
0.40	0.60	0.253	1.960	4.897
0.30	0.70	0.524	1.960	6.172
0.20	0.80	0.842	1.960	7.849
0.10	0.90	1.282	1.960	10.507
0.05	0.95	1.645	1.960	12.995

The calculations that follow are described in more detail by Machin and Campbell (1987).

(a) Comparison of proportions

Suppose we wished to detect a difference in proportions $\delta = \pi_2 - \pi_1$, where $\pi_2 > \pi_1$, with significance level α and power $1 - \beta$. For a χ^2 test without continuity correction, the number in each group should be at least

$$m = (z_\alpha + z_\beta)^2 \{\pi_1(1 - \pi_1) + \pi_2(1 - \pi_2)\}/\delta^2$$

We can also use Figure 8.1, if we require a significance level of 5% and a power of 80%.

Example

In a clinical trial suppose the placebo response is 0.25, and we expect the response to the drug to be 0.50. How many subjects are required in each group so that we have an 80% power at 5% significance level?

$\delta = \pi_2 - \pi_1 = 0.25$, $m = 7.849 \times (0.25 \times 0.75 + 0.5 \times 0.5)/0.25^2 = 54.94$. Thus we need at least 55 patients per group. From Figure 8.1, we would be able to say that the required number of patients is between 50 and 75 per group.

(b) Comparison of means (unpaired data)

Suppose on the control drug we expect the mean response to be μ_1 and on the test we expect it to be μ_2. If the standard deviation, σ, of the response is likely to be the same with both drugs, then for significance level α and power $1 - \beta$ the approximate number of patients per group, is

$$m = \frac{2(z_\alpha + z_\beta)^2 \sigma^2}{\delta^2}, \text{ where } \delta = \mu_2 - \mu_1, \text{ and } \mu_2 > \mu_1$$

Example

Suppose in a clinical trial to reduce blood pressure one wished to detect a difference of 5 mmHg, when the standard deviation of blood pressure is 10 mmHg, with power 90% and 5% significance level.

Here $\delta = 5$, $\sigma = 10$ and $m = 2 \times 10.507 \times 100/25 = 84$ per treatment group.

(c) Comparison of means (paired data)

Suppose in a cross-over trial the anticipated difference between drugs is δ, and this has standard deviation σ. Then with power $1 - \beta$ and significance level α the number of subjects required in the trial is approximately

$$m = \frac{(z_\alpha + z_\beta)^2 \sigma^2}{\delta^2}$$

Example

In a cross-over trial for arthritis, the within-subject anticipated standard deviation of VAS for pain experienced on getting out of bed is $\sigma = 3$ mm. Suppose we wished to detect an improvement in pain scores of 1.5 mm by use of a new drug with power 0.95 and significance level 0.05.

The number of subjects required is $m = 12.995 \times 3^2/1.5^2 = 51.98$. Thus we would need about 52 patients to demonstrate this benefit.

A16 NORMAL PROBABILITY PLOTS

Given a sample $x_1, x_2, \ldots, x_n$, we wish to see if they follow a Normal distribution. To do this:

(1) Rank the data from smallest to largest

$x_{(1)}, x_{(2)}, \ldots, x_{(n)}$

Here $x_{(1)}$ represents the smallest observation and $x_{(n)}$ the largest.
(2) Calculate the corresponding cumulative probability scores $(i - \frac{1}{2})/n$, for $i = 1, 2, \ldots, n$.
(3) From Table T5 compute the Normal ordinates z_i, corresponding to the cumulative probability scores.
(4) Plot the observed values $x_{(i)}$, against the Normal ordinates, z_i. Departures from linearity will indicate a lack of Normality. An estimate of the median is provided by the value of x corresponding to the y of 50%. The inverse of the slope of the fitted line can provide an estimate of the corresponding SD.

Example

The residuals from the regression of FEV_1 on height in Table A14 are 0.12, -0.24, -0.01, -0.06 and 0.18, and we wish to check if these follow a Normal distribution.
Ordered, these become -0.24, -0.06, -0.01, 0.12, 0.18.
The corresponding cumulative probability scores are 0.1, 0.3, 0.5, 0.7, 0.9.
The Normal ordinates z_i are found from Table T5. Thus corresponding to the cumulative probability 0.1, $z = -1.28$, for probability 0.3, $z = -0.52$, and so on, giving -1.28, -0.52, 0.00, 0.52, 1.28 for the five residuals. These are plotted in Figure A1.
We can see that there is no real evidence of a lack of Normality from these data.

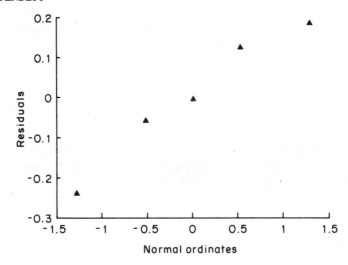

Figure A1   Plot of the residuals calculated from the regression of Table A14 against Normal ordinates

A17 THE KAPLAN–MEIER SURVIVAL CURVE AND THE LOGRANK TEST

These methods are easiest to explain by reference to Table A20. Consider a randomised trial of two treatments A and B, where the outcome is survival time from treatment. Some patients will be lost to follow-up, or will only have been observed for short periods of time and so their observations are *censored*.

Kaplan–Meier survival curves

(1) Order the survival times for both groups combined. Censored observations usually follow death times of the same value.

(2) The number at risk (n_i) is the number of patients alive immediately before event at time t_i.

(3) An event is a death. A censored observation has no associated event.

(4) Calculate the probability of survival from t_{i-1} to t_i as $1 - d_i/n_i$.

(5) The cumulative survival probability is the probability of surviving from 0 up to t_i. It is calculated as

$$(1 - d_i/n_i) \times (1 - d_{i-1}/n_{i-1}) \times \ldots \times (1 - d_1/n_1)$$

(6) Note that a censored observation at time t_i reduces the number at risk by one but does not change the cumulative survival probability at time t_i.

(7) A plot of the cumulative survival probability against t_i, shown in Fig A2, is known as the Kaplan–Meier survival curve.

Table A20 Illustration of calculations for logrank test and Kaplan–Meier survival curve, in a clinical trial of 16 patients

i	Ordered survival time t_i	Treatment	Total number at risk (n_i)	Number of events at time t_i d_i	Probability of survival in t_{i-1}, t_i $1 - d_i/n_i$	Cumulative survival probability	Number at risk in A n_{Ai}	Expected number of events in A e_{Ai}
0	0	—	16	0	1	1	8	0
1	21	A	16	1	0.94	0.94	8	0.5
2	33+	A	15	0	1	0.94	7	0
3	42	B	14	1	0.93	0.87	6	0.43
4	55	A	13	1	0.92	0.80	6	0.46
5	69	A	12	1	0.92	0.74	5	0.42
6	100+	B	11	0	1	0.74	4	0
7	130	A	10	2	0.8	0.59	4	0.80
8	130	A						
9	210	B	8	1	0.875	0.52	2	0.25
10	250+	B	7	0	1	0.52	(See Note 9 in text)	
11	290+	A	6	0	1	0.52		
12	310+	A	5	0	1	0.52		
13	365+	B	4	0	1	0.52		
14	365+	B						
15	365+	B						
16	365+	B						

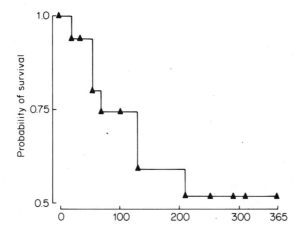

Figure A2   Kaplan–Meier survival curve for data in Table A20

The logrank test

(8) Under the null hypothesis the expected number of events at time t_i is

$$e_{Ai} = (d_{Ai}n_{Ai})/n_i$$

(9) The expected number of events should not be calculated beyond the last event (at time 210 days in this example).

(10) The total number of events expected on A assuming the null hypothesis of no difference between treatments is

$$E_A = \sum e_{Ai}$$

The number expected on B is $E_B = \sum d_i - E_A$.

(11) Calculate

$$\chi^2 = \frac{(O_A - E_A)^2}{E_A} + \frac{(O_B - E_B)^2}{E_B}.$$

This has a χ^2 distribution with df = 1. From Table A20, $O_A = 5$, $O_B = 2$, $E_A = 2.86$, $E_B = 4.14$ and

$$\chi^2 = \frac{(5 - 2.86)^2}{2.86} + \frac{(2 - 4.14)^2}{4.14} = 2.71$$

From Table T3, with df = 1 this gives $p = 0.1$.

Appendix II

Multiple choice questions

Each statement is either true or false.

Chapter 2

(1) In a controlled trial to compare two treatments, the main purpose of randomisation is so that:

    (a) The two groups will be as similar as possible in prognostic factors.
    (b) The clinician does not know which treatment subjects will receive.
    (c) The sample may be referred to a known population.
    (d) The clinician cannot predict in advance which treatment subjects will receive.
    (e) The number of subjects in each treatment group are the same.

(2) Cross-over clinical trials:

    (a) Cannot be randomised.
    (b) Require fewer patients than do comparable parallel clinical trials.
    (c) Are useful in studies involving survival.
    (d) Use the patient as his own control.
    (e) Are usually easier to interpret than the comparable parallel clinical trial.

(3) Cohort studies:

    (a) Are usually more expensive than case-control studies.
    (b) Are not usually used to study rare diseases.
    (c) Provide information on absolute risk.
    (d) Usually concern only a single disease.
    (e) Are rarely subject to bias.

(4)   A case-control study of the suspected association between endometrial carcinoma and oestrogen therapy:

   (a) Can measure the risk to an individual of developing the disease as a result of therapy.
   (b) Will require controls selected randomly from the general population.
   (c) Will require follow-up of a group of women on oestrogen therapy and a control group not on therapy.
   (d) Will not prove that the association, if any, is causal.
   (e) Is unlikely to give biased results because the cases will all have been investigated in hospital.

(5)   In a case-control study of a suspected association between breast cancer and the contraceptive pill:

   (a) The controls should come from the unaffected part of the same population as the cases.
   (b) The controls should exclude women known to be taking the pill at the time of the survey.
   (c) The controls need all to be healthy people.
   (d) The attributable risk of breast cancer resulting from the pill may be directly measured.
   (e) The history of pill-taking in the cases and controls should be assessed by the same criteria.

(6)   When a screening test for disease in asymptomatic patients is used:

   (a) The disease should be rare.
   (b) There should be effective treatment for the disease at an early stage.
   (c) The disease should be accompanied by significant morbidity if left untreated.
   (d) The patients should be a random sample from the population.
   (e) The specificity of the test should be high.

Chapter 3

(7)   In a population presenting to casualty with abdominal pain, 30% of patients have acute appendicitis. 70% of patients with appendicitis have a temperature greater than 37.5°C, 40% of patients without appendicitis have a temperature greater than 37.5°C.

   (a) The sensitivity of temperature greater than 37.5°C as a marker for appendicitis is 21/49.
   (b) The specificity of temperature greater than 37.5°C as a marker for appendicitis is 42/70.
   (c) The predictive value of temperature greater than 37.5°C as a marker for appendicitis is 21/30.
   (d) The predictive value of the test might be different in another population.
   (e) The specificity of the test will depend upon the prevalence of appendicitis in the population to which it is applied.

(8) A new laboratory test is developed for the diagnosis of rectal cancer.

   (a) A sensitivity of 85% implies that 15% of patients with rectal cancer will give negative findings when tested.
   (b) A specificity of 95% implies that 5% of patients with a negative test will actually have rectal cancer.
   (c) A predictive value of 75% implies that 25% of patients with a positive test will not have rectal cancer.
   (d) The sensitivity of the test will depend upon the prevalence of rectal cancer in the population to which it is applied.
   (e) The predictive value of the test will depend upon the prevalence of rectal cancer in the population to which it is applied.

(9) Three tests (A, B and C) for the diagnosis of breast cancer in premenopausal women were assessed against a standard taken to be 100% accurate. Their sensitivities were: A—90%, B—85%, C—80%. Their specificities were: A—100%, B—90%, C—95%. All three tests carried the same cost, and none was associated with any side effects. It follows that:

   (a) In these circumstances test A will always be preferable to test B.
   (b) In these circumstances test B will always be preferable to test C.
   (c) Test B detects a higher proportion of cases than test C.
   (d) There are no false positive results with test A.
   (e) The predictive value of test B will depend on the prevalence of disease in the population to which it is applied.

Chapter 4

(10) The mean of a large sample of size n:

   (a) Is always greater than the median.
   (b) Is calculated from the formula $\sum x/n$.
   (c) Estimates the population mean with greater precision than the mean of a small sample.
   (d) Increases as the sample size increases.
   (e) Is always greater than the standard deviation.

(11) A histogram:

   (a) Usually shows the development of a quantity over time.
   (b) Could be used to show the distribution of lengths of hospital stay in patients admitted with acute asthma.
   (c) Could be used to show the distribution of birth weights in a sample of babies.
   (d) Is the best way to show the relationship between weight and blood pressure in a sample of diabetic patients.
   (e) Conveys information about the spread of a distribution.

(12) The following are measures of the spread of a distribution:

    (a) Interquartile range.
    (b) Standard deviation.
    (c) Range.
    (d) Median.
    (e) Mode.

Chapter 5

(13) The diastolic blood pressures (DBP) of a group of young men are Normally distributed with a mean of 70 mmHg and a standard deviation of 10 mmHg. It follows that:

    (a) About 95% of the men have a DBP between 60 and 80 mmHg.
    (b) About 50% of the men have a DBP above 70 mmHg.
    (c) The distribution of DBP is not skewed.
    (d) All the DBPs must be less than 100 1/min.
    (e) About 2.5% of the men have DBP below 50 mmHg.

(14) Replication of a clinical measurement on the same subject:

    (a) Would show within-observer and between-observer variation are usually equal.
    (b) Is recommended to increase the sample size.
    (c) Would give a complete assessment of its accuracy.
    (d) By two observers is likely to show random, but not systematic, variation.
    (e) Which shows good repeatability indicates that the measurement is valid.

Chapter 6

(15) Following the introduction of a new treatment regimen in an alcohol dependency unit, 'cure' rates improved. The proportion of successful outcomes in the two years following the change was significantly higher than in the preceding two years ($\chi^2_1 = 4.2$, $p < 0.05$). It follows that:

    (a) The probability that the difference or one more extreme occurred by chance is less than 1 in 20.
    (b) The improvement in treatment outcome is clinically important.
    (c) The change in outcome could be due to a confounding factor.
    (d) The new regimen cannot be worse than the old treatment.
    (e) Assuming that there are no biases in the study method, the new treatment should be recommended in preference to the old.

(16) As the size of a random sample increases:

    (a) The standard deviation decreases.
    (b) The standard error of the mean decreases.

(c) The mean decreases.

(d) The range is likely to increase.

(e) The accuracy of the parameter estimates increases.

(17) A 95% confidence interval for a mean:

(a) Is wider than a 99% confidence interval.

(b) In repeated samples will include the population mean 95% of the time.

(c) Will include the sample mean with a probability of 1.

(d) Is a useful way of describing the accuracy of a study.

(e) Will include 95% of the observations of a sample.

(18) In a cross-over clinical trial of two expectorants, 10 patients with chronic coughs were randomly treated with first one and then the other drug, with a washout period in-between. After each drug, they were asked whether the cough was better.

(a) The correct statistical test is Fisher's Exact Test.

(b) The degrees of freedom associated with the appropriate test are 9.

(c) If the result is significant, then the expectorant with the higher cure rate is better.

(d) The numbers are too small to achieve a significant result.

(e) The power of the study is likely to be low.

(19) The p-value:

(a) Is the probability that the null hypothesis is false.

(b) Is large for small studies.

(c) Is the probability of the observed result, or one more extreme, if the null hypothesis were true.

(d) Is $1 -$ type II error.

(e) Can only take a limited number of values such as 0.1, 0.05, 0.01, etc.

Chapter 7

(20) A correlation coefficient:

(a) Always lies in the range 0–1.

(b) Could be used to summarise the relationship between haemoglobin concentration and blood group in a sample of hospital patients.

(c) Could be used to summarise the relationship between mortality from ischaemic heart disease and smoking habit in a case-control study.

(d) Is a measure of the extent to which two continuous variables are linearly related.

(e) Can be used to predict one variable from another.

(21) A linear regression equation:

(a) Is not affected by a change of scale.

(b) Minimises the sum of the differences between the points and the line.

(c) Can be used for prediction.

(d) Might be used to summarise the relationship between forced expiratory volume and age in a cross-sectional study.

(e) Requires that the dependent variable is Normally distributed.

Chapter 8

(22) The number of subjects required in a clinical trial increases as:

(a) The power required increases.
(b) The incidence of disease decreases.
(c) The significance level increases.
(d) The size of the expected treatment effect increased.
(e) The drop-out rate increases.

Chapter 9

(23) In determining whether an observed association is likely to be causal:

(a) The finding should be consistent with the result of other studies.
(b) The absence of a dose–response effect is evidence against causality.
(c) Confounding factors can be ignored.
(d) A significant correlation coefficient between exposure and disease incidence is proof of causality.
(e) Deaths occurring more than 30 years after exposure to the suspected cause are irrelevant.

(24) The prevalence of a disease:

(a) Is the best measure of disease frequency in aetiological studies.
(b) Can only be determined by a cohort study.
(c) Is the number of new cases in a defined population.
(d) Can be standardised for age and sex.
(e) Describes the balance between incidence, mortality and recovery.

(25) The standardised mortality ratio (SMR) for a certain area, with England and Wales as standard, is 50. This means that:

(a) In the year under study, the age-specific death rates in the area were half those in England and Wales.
(b) The population in the area is probably younger than that of England and Wales.
(c) The SMR in the area is half the England and Wales SMR.
(d) Half as many deaths were observed as would have been expected if national age-specific death rates had occurred in the area.
(e) The low death rate in the area cannot be explained simply on the basis of age.

(26) A standardised mortality ratio (SMR) of under 100 from breast cancer in a particular area:

(a) Is statistically significantly different from the standard population.

(b) Indicates a low prevalence of breast cancer in comparison with the standard population.

(c) May indicate a low incidence of breast cancer in comparison with the standard population.

(d) Could be due to the younger age distribution of women in the area.

(e) Could reflect more successful treatment in the area.

General

(27) If systolic blood pressure and racial origin were ascertained in a sample of seven-year-old children selected at random from ten general practice lists:

(a) The distribution of children by racial origin could be illustrated with a bar chart.

(b) The distribution of systolic blood pressures in the children could be illustrated with a histogram.

(c) The relation between systolic blood pressure and racial origin could be summarised by a correlation coefficient.

(d) A regression line could be used to predict systolic blood pressure from racial origin.

(e) Each seven-year-old child on the ten general practice lists had a defined probability of being included in the study sample.

ANSWERS

T = True, F = False

(1) (a) **T**   This is one of the main reasons for randomization. (b) **F**   For this to be true the trial would have to be *blind*. (c) **F**   The comparison is between treatments, not with a known population. (d) **T**   The point being if he knew in advance he might be biased as to whether to admit the patient. (e) **F**   One needs blocked or restricted randomisation to ensure equal numbers.

(2) (a) **F**   The order of administration can be randomised. (b) **T**   Using the patient as his own control means that a separate control group is not required. (c) **F**   They are only of use in studies of chronic disease. (d) **T**   See (b). (e) **F**   If there is a carry-over effect then they can be very difficult to interpret.

(3) (a) **T**   They require large numbers of subjects over long periods. (b) **T**   The numbers involved are usually too great. (c) **T**   The incidence in unexposed subjects can be ascertained. (d) **F**   Cohort studies can be used for a number of diseases. (e) **F**   The 'healthy worker' effect is one bias in cohort studies.

(4) (a) **T**. (b) **F**   The requirement is that controls would have had the same opportunity as the cases of having therapy. (c) **F**   The controls are women who do not have endometrial carcinoma. (d) **T**   Association does not prove causation. (e) **F**   Sources of bias are discussed in Chapter 2.

(5) (a) **T**. (b) **F**   Women taking the pill at the time of the study are also likely to be past users and so this would bias control selection. (c) **F**   This would bias control selection. (d) **F**   The incidence in the unexposed group is not measured in a case-control study. (e) **T**   Otherwise they may be biases between cases and controls

(6) (a) **F**   See section 2.11. (b) **T**   Otherwise it is not worth detecting the disease. (c) **T** Otherwise it is not worth treating. (d) **F**   There is no requirement of a random sample. (e) **T**   Otherwise there will be an unacceptable level of false positives.

(7) Draw up the following 2 × 2 table on 100 subjects.

| | Appendicitis | | |
	Yes	No	Total
Temperature > 37.5°C	21	28	49
Temperature < 37.5°C	9	42	51
Total	30	70	100

The answers follow from the definitions. (a) **F**   21/30. (b) **T**. (c) **F**   21/49. (d) **T**   It depends on the prevalence of the disease. (e) **F**   Specificity is independent of prevalence.

(8) (a) **T**. (b) **F**   Specificity refers to patients without disease. (c) **T**. (d) **F**   Sensitivity is independent of prevalence. (e) **T**   Predictive value is affected by prevalence.

(9) (a) **T**. (b) **F**   In some situations it is better to have a test that is more specific. (c) **F** The proportion of cases detected will depend on the prevalence. (d) **T**. (e) **T**.

(10) (a) **F**   The mean can be greater than the median if the data are positively skewed. (b) **T**. (c) **T**. (d) **F**   The estimate of the mean is not dependent on the sample size. (e) **F** If some of the data are negative the standard deviation can be greater than the mean.

(11) (a) **F**   It usually shows the distribution of a quantity. (b) **T**. (c) **T**. (d) **F**   A scatter plot would be better. (e) **T**.

(12) (a) **T**. (b) **T**. (c) **T**. (d) **F**   The median is a measure of location. (e) **F**   The mode is a measure of location.

(13) (a) **F**   About 68% of the sample lie within those limits. (b) **T**. (c) **T**. (d) **F**   There is a small but non-zero probability that an observation is 3 standard deviations from the mean. (e) **T**.

(14) (a) **F**   There is no requirement that within and between observer variation should be the same. (b) **F**   The sample size is increased by increasing the number of subjects. (c) **F**   The accuracy will depend on having a 'gold standard'. (d) **F**   The observer bias is systematic. (e) **F**   We do not have a measure of bias.

(15) (a) **T**. (b) **F**   Statistical significance is not of clinical importance. (c) **T**. (d) **F**   We

do not know about side effects. (e) **F** We do not know about costs or side effects.

(16) (a) **F** The standard deviation is independent of the sample size. (b) **T**. (c) **F**. (d) **T**. (e) **T**.

(17) (a) **F** A 99% confidence interval is wider than a 95% confidence interval. (b) **T**. (c) **T**. (d) **T**. (e) **F** 2 standard deviations either side of the mean will include about 95% of the observations in the sample.

(18) (a) **F** Fisher's Exact Test does not take into account the paired design. (b) **F** There is one treatment comparison and so one degree of freedom. (c) **F** Significance is not clinical importance. (d) **F** If the difference is very large then the sample big enough. (e) **T** For any realistic sized effect.

(19) (a) **F** See section 6.4. (b) **F** If the treatment effect is large then the p-value might be small. (c) **T**. (d) **F** That is the power. (e) **F** It can take any value between 0 and 1 but is usually quoted for a restricted range.

(20) (a) **F** The range is -1 to 1. (b) **F** Blood group is not continuous. (c) **F** Mortality is not continuous. (d) **T**. (e) **F** The regression equation can be used to predict one variable from another.

(21) (a) **F** The *correlation coefficient* is unaffected by scale changes. (b) **F** It minimises the sum of squares of the differences between the points and the line. (c) **T**. (d) **T**. (e) **F** See section 7.3c.

(22) (a) **T**. (b) **F** The sample size assumes all subjects already have the disease. (c) **F** The sample size increases as the significance level *decreases*. (d) **T**. (e) **T**.

(23) (a) **T**. (b) **T**. (c) **F**. (d) **F** Correlation does not mean causation. (e) **F** Some effects eg exposure to asbestos fibres have a very long latent period.

(24) (a) **F** If the disease has a short duration prevalence may be difficult to measure, and one should measure incidence. (b) **F** One can determine prevalence in a cross-sectional study. (c) **F** That is incidence. (d) **T**. (e) **T**.

(25) (a) **F** It is not necessary for all age-specific rates to be half those of England and Wales—some may be more than half and some less. (b) **F** The SMR adjusts for age. (c) **T**. (d) **T**. (e) **T**.

(26) (a) **F** One would need a mesaure of the standard error to assess statistical significance. (b) **F** Prevalence relates to morbidity not mortality. (c) **T**. (d) **F**. (e) **T**.

(27) (a) **T**. (b) **T**. (c) and (d) **F** Racial origin is not a continuous variable. (e) **T**.

References

Altman, D.G., Gore, S.M., Gardner, M.J. and Pocock, S.J. (1983) Statistical guidelines for contributors to medical journals. *British Medical Journal*, **286**, 1489–1493.

Altman, D.G. and Gardner, M.J. (1988) Confidence intervals for regression and correlation. *British Medical Journal*, **296**, 1238–1242.

Armitage, P.and Berry, G. (1987) *Statistical Methods in Medical Research*, 2nd edition. Oxford: Blackwell.

Armitage, P., Fox, W., Rose, G.A. and Tinker, C.M. (1966) The variability of measurements of casual blood pressure II Survey experience. *Clinical Science*, **30**, 337–344.

Bailar, J.C., Mosteller, F. (1986) *Medical Uses of Statistics*. Massachusetts: N.E.J.M. Books.

Beasley, C.R.W., Rafferty, P. and Holgate, S.T. (1987) Bronchoconstrictor properties of preservatives in ipratopium bromide (Atrovent) nebuliser solution. *British Medical Journal*, **294**, 1197–1198.

Beck, J.R. and Shultz, E.K. (1986) The use of relative operating characteristic (ROC) curves in test performance evaluation. *Archives of Pathology and Laboratory Medicine*, **110**, 13–20.

Begg, C.B. (1987) Biases in the assessment of diagnostic tests. *Statistics in Medicine*, **6**, 411–423.

Bell, B.A., Smith, M.A., Kean, D.M. *et al.* (1987) Brain water measured by magnetic resonance imaging. *Lancet*, **i**, 66–68.

Belsey, R., Goitein, R.K. and Baer, D.M. (1987) Evaluation of a laboratory system intended for use in physicians' offices. I. Reliability of results produced by trained laboratory technologists. *Journal of the American Medical Association*, **258**, 353–356.

Beral, V., Fraser, P. and Chilvers, C.E.D. (1978) Does pregnancy protect against ovarian cancer? *Lancet*, **i**, 1083–1087.

Bland, M. (1987) An Introduction to Medical Statistics. Oxford: Oxford University Press.

Bland, J.M. and Altman, D.G. (1986) Statistical methods for assessing agreement between two methods of clinical measurement. *Lancet*, **i**, 307–310.

Bourke, G.J., Daly, L.E. and McGilvray, J. (1985) *Interpretation and Uses of Medical Statistics*. Oxford: Blackwell Scientific.

Brown, L.M., Pottern, L.M. and Hoover, R.N. (1987) Testicular cancer in young men: the search for causes of the epidemic increase in the United States. *British Journal of Epidemiology and Community Health*, **41**, 349–354.

Burke, D. and Yiamouyannis, J. (1975) Letters to Hon. James Delany. *Congressional Record*, **191**, H7172–7176 and H12731–12734.

Campbell, M.J. (1985) Predicting running speed from a simple questionnaire. *British Journal of Sports Medicine*, **19**, 142–144.

Campbell, M.J. and Gardner, M.J. (1988) Calculating confidence intervals for some non-parametric tests. *British Medical Journal*, **296**, 1454–1456.

Campbell, M.J. and Williams, J.D. (1989) Comparison of methods (letter). *Respiratory Medicine*, **83**, 167–169.

Campbell, M.J., Browne, D., Waters, W.E. (1985) Can general practioners influence exercise ? Controlled trial. *British Medical Journal*, **290**, 1044–1046.

Campbell, M.J., Lewry, J. and Wailoo, M. (1988) Further evidence for the effect of passive smoking on neonates. *Postgraduate Medical Journal*, **64**, 663–665.

Campbell, M.J., Elwood, P.C., Mackean, J. and Waters, W.E. (1985) Mortality, haemoglobin level and haematocrit in women. *Journal of Chronic Diseases*, **38**, 881–889.

Campbell, H., Byass, P., Lamont, A.C., Forgie, I.M., O'Neill, K.P., Lloyd-Evans, N. and Greenwood, B.M. (1989) Assessment of clinical criteria for identification of severe acute lower respiratory tract infections in children. *Lancet*, **i**, 297–299.

Chant, A.D.B, Turner, D.T.L. and Machin, D. (1984) Metionidazole *v* ampicillin: differing effects on the postoperative recovery. *Annals of the Royal College of Surgeons of England*, **66**, 96–97.

Christie, D. (1979) Before and after comparisons: a cautionary tale. *British Medical Journal*, **279**, 1629–1630.

Cohen, D., Dodds, R. and Viberti, G. (1987) Effect of protein restriction in insulin dependent diabetics at risk of nephropathy. *British Medical Journal*, **294**, 795–797.

Colton, T. (1974) *Statistics in Medicine*. Boston: Little Brown.

Conover, W.J. (1980) *Practical Non-Parametric Statistics*. New York: Wiley.

Doll, R. and Hill, A.B. (1964) Mortality in relation to smoking: ten years' observation of British doctors. *British Medical Journal*, **1**, 1399–1410, 1460–1467.

Dowson, D.I., Lewith, G.T. and Machin, D. (1985) The affects of acupuncture versus placebo in the treatment of headache. *Pain*, **23**, 35–42.

Elwood, P.C. and Sweetnam, P.M. (1979) Aspirin and secondary mortality after myocardial infarction. *Lancet*, **ii**, 1313–1315.

Emerson, J.D. and Colditz, G.A. (1983) Use of statistical analysis in the New England Journal of Medicine. *New England Journal of Medicine*, **309**, 709–713.

Familiari, L., Postorino, S., Turiano, S. and Luzza, G. (1981) Comparison of pirenzepine and trithiozine with placebo in treatment of peptic ulcer. *Clinical Trial Journal*, **18**, 363–368.

Feinstein, A.R. (1987) Quantitative ambiguities in matched versus unmatched analyses of the 2×2 table for a case-control study. *International Journal of Epidemiology*, **16**, 128–13.

Findlay, I.N., Taylor, R.S., Dargie, H.J. *et al.* (1987) Cardiovascular effects of training for a marathon run in unfit middle-aged men. *Brititish Medical Journal*, **295**, 521–524.

Fraser, C.G. and Fogarty, Y. (1989) Interpreting laboratory results. *British Medical Journal*, **298**, 1659–60.

Frazer, M.I., Sutherst, J.R. and Holland, E.F.N. (1987) Visual analogue scores and urinary incontinence. *British Medical Journal*, **295**, 582.

Gardner, M.J. and Altman, D.G. (1989) *Statistics with Confidence*. London: British Medical Association.

Gardner, M.J., Machin, D. and Campbell, M.J. (1986) Use of checklists for the assessment of the statistical content of medical studies. *British Medical Journal*, **292**, 810–812.

Gatling, W., Mullee, M.A. and Hill, R.D. (1988) The prevalence of proteinuria detected by Albustix in a defined diabetic population. *Diabetic Medicine*, **5**, 256–260.

Godfrey, K. (1985) Simple linear regression in medical research. *New England Journal of Medicine*, **313**, 1629–1636.

Gore, S.M. and Altman, D.G. (1982) *Statistics in Practice*. London: British Medical Association.

Hannequin, P., Liehn, J.C., Maes, B. and Delisle, M.J. (1988) Multivariate analysis in solitary cold thyroid nodules for the diagnosis of malignancy. *European Journal of Cancer and Clinical Oncology*, **24**, 881–888.

Hindmarsh, P.C. and Brook, C.G.D. (1987) Effect of growth hormone on short normal children. *British Medical Journal*, **295**, 573–577.

Horwitz, R.I. and Feinstein, A.R. (1978) Alternative analytic methods for case-control studies of estrogens and endometrial cancer. *New England Journal of Medicine*, **299**, 1089–1094.

Jung, K., Perganda, M., Schimke, E., Ratzmann, K.P. and Ilius, A. (1988) Urinary enzymes and low-molecular-mass proteins as indicators of diabetic nephropathy. *Clinical Chemistry*, **34**, 544–547.

Knill-Jones, R.P. (1987) Diagnostic systems as an aid to clinical decision making. *British Medical Journal*, **295**, 1392–1396.

Last, R.J. (1987) Accumulating evidence from independent studies. What we can win and what we can lose. *Statistics in Medicine*, **6**, 221–228.

Larochelle, P., Cusson, J.R., Gutkowska, J., Schiffrin, E.L., Hamet, P., Kuchel, O., Genest, J. and Cantin, M. (1987) Plasma atrial natriuretic factor concentrations in essential and renovascular hypertension. *British Medical Journal*, **294**, 1249–1252.

Lindley, D.V. and Scott, W.F. (1984) *New Cambridge Elementary Statistical Tables*. Cambridge: Cambridge University Press.

Loirat, P., Rohan, J., Baillet, A., Beaufils, F., David, R. and Chapman, A. (1978) Increased glomerular filtration rate in patients with major burns and its effect on the pharmacokinetics of tobramycin. *New England Journal of Medicine*, **299**, 915–919.

Macartney, F.J. (1987) Diagnostic logic. *British Medical Journal*, **295**, 1325–1331.

Machin, D. and Campbell, M.J. (1987) *Statistical Tables for the Design of Clinical Trials*. Oxford: Blackwell Scientific Publications.

Machin, D., Lewith, G.T. and Wylson, S. (1988) Pain measurement in randomized clinical trials: A comparison of two pain scales. *Clinical Journal of Pain*, **4**, 161–168.

McIllmurray, M.B. and Turkie, W. (1987) Controlled trial of γ-linolenic acid in Dukes's C colorectal cancer. *British Medical Journal*, **294**, 1260 and **295**, 475.

McMaster, V., Nichols, S. and Machin, D. (1985) Evaluation of breast self-examination teaching materials in a primary care setting. *Journal of the Royal College of General Practitioners*, **35**, 578–580.

Mills, S., Campbell, M.J. and Waters, W.E. (1986) Public knowledge of AIDS and the DHSS advertisement campaign. *British Medical Journal*, **293**, 1089–1090.

Milsom, S., Ibbertson, K., Hannan, S., Shaw, D. and Pybus, J. (1987) Simple test of intestinal calcium absorption measured by stable strontium. *British Medical Journal*, **295**, 231–234.

Morris, J.A. and Gardner, M.J. (1988) Calculating confidence intervals for relative risks (odds ratios) and standardised ratios and rates. *British Medical Journal*, **296**, 1313–1316.

Moser, C.A. and Kalton, G. (1971) *Survey Methods in Social Investigation*. Aldershot: Gower Publishing Company Ltd.

Mountain, R., Zwillich, C. and Weil, J. (1978) Hypoventilation in obstructive lung disease: the role of familial factors. *New England Journal of Medicine*, **298**, 521–525.

Musk, A.W., Cotes, J.E., Bevan, C. and Campbell, M.J. (1981) Relationship between type of simple coalworkers' pneumoconiosis and lung function. A nine-year follow-up study of subjects with small rounded opacities. *British Journal of Industrial Medicine*, **38**, 313–320.

Myers, E.R., Sondheimer, S.J., Freeman, E.W., Strauss, J.F. and Rickels, K. (1987) Serum progesterone levels following vaginal administration of progesterone during the luteal phase. *Fertility and Sterility*, **47**, 71–75.

Nichols, S., Koch, E., Lallemand, R.J., Izzard, L., Machin, D. and Mullee, M.A. (1986) Randomised trial of compliance with screening for colorectal cancer. *British Medical Journal*, **293**, 107–110.

Oldham, P.D. (1968) *Measurement in Medicine*. London: English Universities Press.

Oldham, P.D. and Newell, D.J. (1977) Fluoridation of water supplies and cancer—a possible association? *Applied Statistics*, **26**, 125–135.

Oleinick, M.S., Bahn, A.K. and Eisenberg, L. (1966) Early socialization experiences and intrafamilial environment. A study of psychiatric outpatient and control group children. *Archives of General Psychiatry*, **15**, 344–347.

Olsen, M., Petring, O.U. and Rossing, N. (1987) Exaggerated postural vasoconstrictor reflex in Raynaud's phenomenon. *British Medical Journal*, **294**, 1186–1188.

Parker, S.G. and Kassiver, J.P. (1987) Decision analysis. *New England Journal of Medicine*, **316**, 250–258.

Persantine–Aspirin Reinfarction Study Research Group (1980) Persantine and aspirin in coronary heart disease. *Circulation*, **62**, 449–461.

Piedras, J., Cordon, S., Perez-Toval, C., Lince, E. and Gorba-Flores, J. (1983) Predictive value of serum ferritin in anaemia development after insertion of TCu220 Intrauterine device. *Contraception*, **27**, 289–297.

Pocock, S.J. (1983) *Clinical Trials: A Practical Approach*. Chichester: Wiley.

Powell-Tuck, J., Macrae, K.D., Healy, M.J.R., Lennard-Jones, J.E. and Parkins, R.A. (1986) A defence of the small clinical trial: evaluation of three gastroenterological studies. *British Medical Journal*, **292**, 599–602.

Rothman, K. (1986) *Modern Epidemiology*. Boston: Little, Brown & Co.

Royal College of General Practitioners (1981) Breast cancer and oral contraceptives. *British Medical Journal*, **282**, 2089–2093.

Royal College of Physicians (1983) *Health or Smoking?* London: Pitman.

Royal College of General Practitioners (1981) Further analysis of mortality in oral contraceptive users. *Lancet*, **i**, 541–46.

Sampson, G.A. and Prescott, P. (1981) The assessment of the symptoms of premenstrual syndrome and their response to therapy. *British Journal of Psychiatry*, **138**, 399–405.

Schatzkin, A., Jones, Y., Hoover, R.N. *et al.* (1987) Alcohol consumption and breast cancer in the epidemiologic follow-up study of the first national health and nutrition examination survey. *New England Journal of Medicine*, **316**, 1169–1173.

Scott, R.S., Knowles, R.L. and Beaver, D.W. (1984) Treatment of poorly controlled non-insulin-dependent diabetic patients with acarbose. *Australian and New Zealand Journal of Medicine*, **14**, 649–654.

Schwartz, D., Flamant, R. and Lellouch, J. (1980) *Clinical Trials* (trans. M.J.R. Healy). London: Academic Press.

Sherry, B., Jack, R.M., Weber, A. and Smith, A.L. (1988) Reference interval for prealbumin for children 2 to 36 months old. *Clinical Chemistry*, **34**, 1878–1880.

Sleep, J. and Grant, A. (1987) West Berkshire perineal management trial: three year follow up. *British Medical Journal*, **295**, 749–751.

Smith, G. and Waters, W.E. (1983) An epidemiological study of factors associated with perimenopausal hot flushes. *Public Health*, **97**, 347–351.

Snedecor, G.W. and Cochran, W.G. (1980) *Statistical Methods*, 6th edition. Ames: Iowa State University Press.

Soothill, P.W., Nicolcaides, K.H. and Campbell, S. (1987) Prenatal asphyxia, hyperlacticaemia, hypoglycaemia, and erythroblastosis in growth retarded fetuses. *British Medical Journal*, **294**, 1051–1053.

Strike, P.W. (1981) *Medical Laboratory Statistics*. Bristol: Wright.

Sutton, R., Campbell, M.J., Cooke, T., Nicholson, R., Griffiths, K. and Taylor, I. (1987) Predictive power of progesterone receptor status in early breast carcinoma. *British Journal of Surgery*, **74**, 223–226.

Tango, T. (1986) Estimation of normal ranges of clinical laboratory data. *Statistics in Medicine*, **5**, 335–346.

Thakur, C.P., Sharma, R.N. and Akhtar, H.S.M.Q. (1981) Full moon and poisoning. *British Medical Journal*, **281**, 1684.

Thomas, K.B. (1987) General practice consultations: Is there any point in being positive? *British Medical Journal*, **294**, 1200–1202.

Tippett, P.A., Dennis, N.R., Machin, D., Price, C.P. and Clayton, B.E. (1982) Creatinine kinase activity in the detection of carriers of Duchenne muscular dystrophy: comparison of two methods. *Clinica Chimica Acta*, **121**, 345–359.

Vessey, M., Baron J, Doll R, McPherson, K. and Yeates, D. (1983) Oral contraceptives and breast cancer: Final report of an epidemiological study. *British Journal of Cancer*, **47**, 455–462.

Waters, W.E. (1971) Migraine: intelligence, social class and familial prevalence. *British Medical Journal*, **2**, 77–81.

Weiner, D.A., Ryan, T.J., McCabe, C.H. *et al.* (1979) Exercise stress testing. Correlations among history of angina, ST segment response and prevalence of coronary artery disease in the coronary artery surgery study (CASS). *New England Journal of Medicine*, **301**, 230–235.

Whitehead, J. (1983) *The Design and Analysis of Sequential Clinical Trials*. Chichester: Ellis Horwood.

Wynne, G., Marteau, T.M., Johnson, M., Whiteley, C.A. and Evans, T.R. (1987) Inability of trained nurses to perform basic life support. *British Medical Journal*, **294**, 1198–1199.

Statistical tables

Table T1 The Normal distribution
The value tabulated is the probability, α, that a random variable, Normally distributed with mean zero and standard deviation one will be greater than z or less than $-z$.

z	0.00	0.01	0.02	0.03	0.04	0.05	0.06	0.07	0.08	0.09
0.00	1.0000	0.9920	0.9840	0.9761	0.9681	0.9601	0.9522	0.9442	0.9362	0.9283
0.10	0.9203	0.9124	0.9045	0.8966	0.8887	0.8808	0.8729	0.8650	0.8572	0.8493
0.20	0.8415	0.8337	0.8259	0.8181	0.8103	0.8026	0.7949	0.7872	0.7795	0.7718
0.30	0.7642	0.7566	0.7490	0.7414	0.7339	0.7263	0.7188	0.7114	0.7039	0.6965
0.40	0.6892	0.6818	0.6745	0.6672	0.6599	0.6527	0.6455	0.6384	0.6312	0.6241
0.50	0.6171	0.6101	0.6031	0.5961	0.5892	0.5823	0.5755	0.5687	0.5619	0.5552
0.60	0.5485	0.5419	0.5353	0.5287	0.5222	0.5157	0.5093	0.5029	0.4965	0.4902
0.70	0.4839	0.4777	0.4715	0.4654	0.4593	0.4533	0.4473	0.4413	0.4354	0.4295
0.80	0.4237	0.4179	0.4122	0.4065	0.4009	0.3953	0.3898	0.3843	0.3789	0.3735
0.90	0.3681	0.3628	0.3576	0.3524	0.3472	0.3421	0.3371	0.3320	0.3271	0.3222
0.00	0.3173	0.3125	0.3077	0.3030	0.2983	0.2937	0.2891	0.2846	0.2801	0.2757

z	0.00	0.01	0.02	0.03	0.04	0.05	0.06	0.07	0.08	0.09
1.00	0.3173	0.3125	0.3077	0.3030	0.2983	0.2937	0.2891	0.2846	0.2801	0.2757
1.10	0.2713	0.2670	0.2627	0.2585	0.2543	0.2501	0.2460	0.2420	0.2380	0.2340
1.20	0.2301	0.2263	0.2225	0.2187	0.2150	0.2113	0.2077	0.2041	0.2005	0.1971
1.30	0.1936	0.1902	0.1868	0.1835	0.1802	0.1770	0.1738	0.1707	0.1676	0.1645
1.40	0.1615	0.1585	0.1556	0.1527	0.1499	0.1471	0.1443	0.1416	0.1389	0.1362
1.50	0.1336	0.1310	0.1285	0.1260	0.1236	0.1211	0.1188	0.1164	0.1141	0.1118
1.60	0.1096	0.1074	0.1052	0.1031	0.1010	0.0989	0.0969	0.0949	0.0930	0.0910
1.70	0.0891	0.0873	0.0854	0.0836	0.0819	0.0801	0.0784	0.0767	0.0751	0.0735
1.80	0.0719	0.0703	0.0688	0.0672	0.0658	0.0643	0.0629	0.0615	0.0601	0.0588
1.90	0.0574	0.0561	0.0549	0.0536	0.0524	0.0512	0.0500	0.0488	0.0477	0.0466
2.00	0.0455	0.0444	0.0434	0.0424	0.0414	0.0404	0.0394	0.0385	0.0375	0.0366

z	0.00	0.01	0.02	0.03	0.04	0.05	0.06	0.07	0.08	0.09
2.00	0.0455	0.0444	0.0434	0.0424	0.0414	0.0404	0.0394	0.0385	0.0375	0.0366
2.10	0.0357	0.0349	0.0340	0.0332	0.0324	0.0316	0.0308	0.0300	0.0293	0.0285
2.20	0.0278	0.0271	0.0264	0.0257	0.0251	0.0244	0.0238	0.0232	0.0226	0.0220
2.30	0.0214	0.0209	0.0203	0.0198	0.0193	0.0188	0.0183	0.0178	0.0173	0.0168
2.40	0.0164	0.0160	0.0155	0.0151	0.0147	0.0143	0.0139	0.0135	0.0131	0.0128
2.50	0.0124	0.0121	0.0117	0.0114	0.0111	0.0108	0.0105	0.0102	0.0099	0.0096
2.60	0.0093	0.0091	0.0088	0.0085	0.0083	0.0080	0.0078	0.0076	0.0074	0.0071
2.70	0.0069	0.0067	0.0065	0.0063	0.0061	0.0060	0.0058	0.0056	0.0054	0.0053
2.80	0.0051	0.0050	0.0048	0.0047	0.0045	0.0044	0.0042	0.0041	0.0040	0.0039
2.90	0.0037	0.0036	0.0035	0.0034	0.0033	0.0032	0.0031	0.0030	0.0029	0.0028
3.00	0.0027	0.0026	0.0025	0.0024	0.0024	0.0023	0.0022	0.0021	0.0021	0.0020

Table T2 Student's t-distribution

The value tabulated is t_α, such that if X is distributed as Student's t-distribution with df degrees of freedom, then α is the probability that $X \leq -t_\alpha$ or $X \geq t_\alpha$.

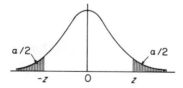

df	\(\alpha \)							
	0.200	0.100	0.050	0.040	0.030	0.020	0.010	0.001
1	3.078	6.314	12.706	15.895	21.205	31.821	63.657	636.6
2	1.886	2.920	4.303	5.512	6.811	6.965	9.925	31.60
3	1.634	2.353	3.182	3.562	4.032	4.541	5.842	12.92
4	1.530	2.132	2.776	3.007	3.319	3.747	4.604	8.610
5	1.474	2.015	2.571	2.745	2.996	3.365	4.032	6.869
6	1.439	1.943	2.447	2.594	2.812	3.143	3.707	5.959
7	1.414	1.895	2.365	2.495	2.693	2.998	3.499	5.408
8	1.397	1.860	2.306	2.426	2.610	2.896	3.355	5.041
9	1.383	1.833	2.262	2.374	2.549	2.821	3.250	4.781
10	1.372	1.812	2.228	2.334	2.502	2.764	3.169	4.587
11	1.363	1.796	2.201	2.303	2.465	2.718	3.106	4.437
12	1.356	1.782	2.179	2.277	2.434	2.681	3.055	4.318
13	1.350	1.771	2.160	2.256	2.409	2.650	2.012	4.221
14	1.345	1.761	2.145	2.238	2.388	2.624	2.977	4.140
15	1.340	1.753	2.131	2.222	2.370	2.602	2.947	4.073
16	1.337	1.746	2.120	2.209	2.355	2.583	2.921	4.015
17	1.333	1.740	2.110	2.198	2.341	2.567	2.898	3.965
18	1.330	1.734	2.101	2.187	2.329	2.552	2.878	3.922
19	1.328	1.729	2.093	2.178	2.319	2.539	2.861	3.883
20	1.325	1.725	2.086	2.170	2.309	2.528	2.845	3.850
∞	1.282	1.645	1.960	2.054	2.170	2.326	2.576	3.291

Table T3 The χ^2 distribution

The value tabulated is $\chi^2(\alpha)$, such that if X is distributed as χ^2 with df degrees of freedom, then α is the probability that $X \geq \chi^2$.

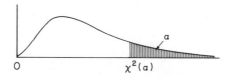

df	α							
	0.200	0.100	0.050	0.040	0.030	0.020	0.010	0.001
1	1.64	2.71	3.84	4.22	4.71	5.41	6.63	10.83
2	3.22	4.61	5.99	6.44	7.01	7.82	9.21	13.82
3	4.64	6.25	7.81	8.31	8.95	9.84	11.34	16.27
4	5.99	7.78	9.49	10.03	10.71	11.67	13.28	18.47
5	7.29	9.24	11.07	11.64	12.37	13.39	15.09	20.52
6	8.56	10.64	12.59	13.20	13.97	15.03	16.81	22.46
7	9.80	12.02	14.07	14.70	15.51	16.62	18.48	24.32
8	11.03	13.36	15.51	16.17	17.01	18.17	20.09	26.13
9	12.24	14.68	16.92	17.61	18.48	19.68	21.67	27.88
10	13.44	15.99	18.31	19.02	19.92	21.16	23.21	29.59
11	14.63	17.28	19.68	20.41	21.34	22.62	24.73	31.26
12	15.81	18.55	21.03	21.79	22.74	24.05	26.22	32.91
13	16.98	19.81	22.36	23.14	24.12	25.47	27.69	34.53
14	18.15	21.06	23.68	24.49	25.49	26.87	29.14	36.12
15	19.31	22.31	25.00	25.82	26.85	28.26	30.58	37.70
16	20.47	23.54	26.30	27.14	28.19	29.63	32.00	39.25
17	21.61	24.77	27.59	28.45	29.52	31.00	33.41	40.79
18	22.76	25.99	28.87	29.75	30.84	32.35	34.81	42.31
19	23.90	27.20	30.14	31.04	32.16	33.69	36.19	43.82
20	25.04	28.41	31.41	32.32	33.46	35.02	37.57	45.32

Table T4   Random numbers
Each digit is equally likely to appear and cannot be predicted from any combination of other digits.

75792	78245	83270	59987	75253	42729	98917	83137	67588	93846
80169	88847	36686	36601	91654	44249	52586	25702	09575	18939
94071	63090	23901	93268	53316	87773	89260	04804	99479	83909
67970	29162	60224	61042	98324	30425	37677	90382	96230	84565
91577	43019	67511	28527	61750	55267	07847	50165	26793	80918
84334	54827	51955	47256	21387	28456	77296	41283	01482	44494
03778	05031	90146	59031	96758	57420	23581	38824	49592	18593
58563	84810	22446	80149	99676	83102	35381	94030	59560	32145
29068	74625	90665	52747	09364	57491	59049	19767	83081	78441
90047	44763	44534	55425	67170	67937	88962	49992	53583	37864
54870	35009	84524	32309	88815	86792	89097	66600	26195	88326
23327	78957	50987	77876	63960	53986	46771	80998	95229	59606
03876	89100	66895	89468	96684	95491	32222	58708	34408	66930
14846	86619	04238	36182	05294	43791	88149	22637	56775	52091
94731	63786	88290	60990	98407	43437	74233	25880	96898	52186
96046	51589	84509	98162	39162	59469	60563	74917	02413	17967
95188	25011	29947	48896	83408	79684	11353	13636	46380	69003
67416	00626	49781	77833	47073	59147	50469	10807	58985	98881
50002	97121	26652	23667	13819	54138	54173	69234	28657	01031
50806	62492	67131	02610	43964	19528	68333	69484	23527	96974
43619	79413	45456	31642	78162	81686	73687	19751	24727	98742
90476	58785	15177	81377	26671	70548	41383	59773	59835	13719
43241	22852	28915	49692	75981	74215	65915	36489	10233	89897
57434	86821	63717	54640	28782	24046	84755	83021	85436	29813
15731	12986	03008	18739	07726	75512	65295	15089	81094	05260
34706	04386	02945	72555	97249	16798	05643	42343	36106	63948
16759	74867	62702	32840	08565	18403	10421	60687	68599	78034
11895	74173	72423	62838	89382	57437	85314	75320	01988	52518
87597	21289	30904	13209	04244	53651	28373	90759	70286	49678
63656	28328	25428	38671	97372	69256	49364	35398	30808	59082
72414	71686	65513	81236	26205	10013	80610	40509	50045	70530
69337	19016	50420	38803	55793	84035	93051	57693	33673	67434
64310	62819	20242	08632	83905	49477	29409	96563	86993	91207
31243	63913	66340	91169	28560	69220	14730	19752	51636	59434
39951	83556	88718	68802	06170	90451	58926	50125	28532	17189
57473	53613	76478	82668	28315	05975	96324	96135	14255	29991
50259	80588	94408	55754	79166	20490	97112	25904	20254	08781
48449	97696	14321	92549	95812	78371	77678	56618	44769	57413
50830	52921	41365	46257	66889	29420	95250	24080	08600	04189
94646	37630	50246	53925	95496	82773	41021	95435	83812	52558
49344	07037	24221	41955	47211	43418	45703	78779	77215	44594
49201	66377	64188	50398	33157	87375	55885	14174	03105	85821
57221	54927	59025	46847	35894	14639	38452	89166	72843	40954
65391	57289	67771	99160	08184	26262	46577	32603	21677	54104
01029	99783	63250	39198	51042	36834	40450	90864	49953	61032
23218	67476	45675	17299	85685	57294	30847	39985	44402	76665
35175	51935	85800	91083	97112	20865	96101	83276	84149	11443
28442	12188	99908	51660	34350	66572	43047	30217	44491	79042
89327	26880	83020	20428	87554	33251	80684	01964	04106	28243

Table T5   Normal ordinates for cumulative probabilities
The value tabulated is z such that for a given probability α, a random variable, Normally distributed
with mean zero and standard deviation one will be less than z with probability α.

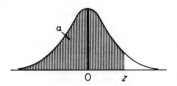

	α									
	0.01	0.01	0.02	0.03	0.04	0.05	0.06	0.07	0.08	0.09
0.00	–	−2.33	−2.05	−1.88	−1.75	−1.64	−1.56	−1.48	−1.41	−1.34
0.10	−1.28	−1.23	−1.17	−1.13	−1.08	−1.04	−0.99	−0.95	−0.92	−0.88
0.20	−0.84	−0.81	−0.77	−0.74	−0.71	−0.67	−0.64	−0.61	−0.58	−0.55
0.30	−0.52	−0.50	−0.47	−0.44	−0.41	−0.39	−0.36	−0.33	−0.31	−0.28
0.40	−0.25	−0.23	−0.20	−0.18	−0.15	−0.13	−0.10	−0.08	−0.05	−0.03
0.50	0.00	0.03	0.05	0.08	0.10	0.13	0.15	0.18	0.20	0.23
0.60	0.25	0.28	0.31	0.33	0.36	0.39	0.41	0.44	0.47	0.50
0.70	0.52	0.55	0.58	0.61	0.64	0.67	0.71	0.74	0.77	0.81
0.80	0.84	0.88	0.92	0.95	0.99	1.04	1.08	1.13	1.17	1.23
0.90	1.28	1.34	1.41	1.48	1.56	1.64	1.75	1.88	2.05	2.33

Index